Redescribing Bioethics

Revolutionary Bioethics

Series Editor: Rachel Haliburton, University of Sudbury

Revolutionary Bioethics is a new series composed of scholarly monographs and edited collections organized around specific topics that explore bioethical theory and practice through the frameworks provided by feminist ethics, narrative ethics, and virtue ethics, challenging the assumptions of mainstream bioethics in the process. Contemporary mainstream bioethics has become ideological and repetitive, a defender of activities that bioethics was originally created to critique, and an apologist for unethical practices and policies in medicine that it once saw itself as fighting against. Taking its title from recent work being done on MacIntyre's neo-Aristotelian ethics, Revolutionary Bioethics is organized around the idea that bioethics needs to reform both its theory and practice, and its goal is to begin the conversation about what a transformed bioethics—one that is unafraid to explore new theoretical approaches, and to examine and critique current bioethical practices—might look like.

Titles in the Series

Redescribing Bioethics: How the Field Constructs Its Argument, by Tod S. Chambers
Righting Health Policy: Bioethics, Political Philosophy, and the Normative Justification of Health Law and Policy, by D. Robert MacDougall
Caregiving, Carebots, and Contagion, by Michael C. Brannigan
Engineering Perfection: Solidarity, Disability, and Well-being, by Elyse Purcell
Physician-Assisted Suicide and Euthanasia: Before, During, and After the Third Reich, edited by Sheldon Rubenfeld and Daniel P. Sulmasy, with Astrid Ley

Redescribing Bioethics

How the Field Constructs Its Argument

Tod S. Chambers

LEXINGTON BOOKS
Lanham • Boulder • New York • London

Published by Lexington Books
An imprint of The Rowman & Littlefield Publishing Group, Inc.
4501 Forbes Boulevard, Suite 200, Lanham, Maryland 20706
www.rowman.com

86-90 Paul Street, London EC2A 4NE

British Library Cataloguing in Publication Information Available

Library of Congress Cataloging-in-Publication Data

Names: Chambers, Tod, author.
Title: Redescribing bioethics : how the field constructs its argument / Tod S. Chambers.
Description: Lanham : Lexington Books, [2025] | Series: Revolutionary bioethics | Includes bibliographical references and index.
Identifiers: LCCN 2024038585 (print) | LCCN 2024038586 (ebook) | ISBN 9781666924442 (cloth) | ISBN 9781666924459 (epub)
Subjects: LCSH: Bioethics.
Classification: LCC QH332 .C45 2025 (print) | LCC QH332 (ebook) | DDC 174.2–dc23/eng/20241030
LC record available at https://lccn.loc.gov/2024038585
LC ebook record available at https://lccn.loc.gov/2024038586

∞™ The paper used in this publication meets the minimum requirements of American National Standard for Information Sciences—Permanence of Paper for Printed Library Materials, ANSI/NISO Z39.48-1992.

To my children who have both been redescribing themselves since they were born.

Contents

Acknowledgments

First and foremost, I wish to acknowledge the extraordinary support that I have received from the large number of amazing colleagues, past and current, who have been with me at Northwestern University in Chicago, IL. In both formal presentations and informal discussions, many of the ideas in this book were developed through their assistance: Jim Bresnehan, Kathryn Montgomery, Mark Sheldon, Katie Watson, Alice Dreger, Catherine Belling, Sarah Rodgriguez, Megan Crowley-Matoka, Les Friedman, Gretchen Case, Joel Frader, Laurie Zoloth, Debjani Murkerjee, John Franklin, Lisa Campo-Engelstein, Kristi Kirschner, and Ray Curry. Parts of this book were written when I was a member of the Institute for Advanced Study in Princeton, NJ. I am particularly indebted to Carl Elliott, Leigh Turner, Ray De Vries, Trudo Lemmens, Joe Davis, Chuck Bosk, and Louis Charland, all of whom were also members during that year. I also have a debt to a large number of scholars in bioethics and medical humanities who have either read versions of the work or heard presentations, although they may not have agreed with any of the ideas. Of the many, I would like to thank Martha Montello, Rita Charon, Hilde Lindemann, Larry Churchill, Judith Andre, Howard Brody, Anne Hawkins, Bob Baker, John Lantos, Ronald Carson, Micah Hester, Tom Buller, Mark Kuzckweski, Kayhan Parsi, Anne Hudson Jones, Suzanne Poirier, Jamie Nelson, Tess Jones, Bernice Hauseman, Autumn Fiester, and Tyler Tate. I also wish to express special thanks to Anna Fenton Hathaway, who as a freelance editor and literature scholar makes me appear a better writer and thinker than I actually am. And finally, to my wife Megan Shanks, who kindly continues to pretend to be interested in what I am working on.

Parts of chapter 1 originally appeared as "Retrodiction and the Histories of Bioethics," *Medical Humanities Review* 12, no. 1 (1998): 9–22 and parts of chapter 5 as "Root Metaphor and Bioethics," *Perspectives in Biology and Medicine* 59, no. 3 (2016): 311–325. I wish to thank the journals for giving permission for these essays to be reprinted.

Introduction

Describing the World

It is often noted that at the beginning of the development of bioethics as an academic field, many of the most prominent voices were those of theologians. Two leading theologians engaged in the field at that time were Joseph Fletcher and Paul Ramsey. While the two shared a Protestant background—Fletcher was Episcopalian and Ramsey was Methodist—they often found themselves on opposite ends of the field's debates.[1] One of these debates was over biomedical assistance in human reproduction, or, to be more specific, interventions such as genetic manipulation, cloning, and artificial insemination through a donor.

In his discussion of artificial insemination in *Fabricated Man* (1974), Ramsey begins with a reference to a classic dystopia novel: "Aldous Huxley's fertilizing and decanting rooms in the Central London Hatchery (*Brave New World*) will become a possibility within the next fifteen to fifty years."[2] Here and throughout, Ramsey portrays this possibility as a "breach" of an essential aspect of what it means to be human, as it bypasses the traditional understanding of parenthood. His description of artificial insemination is filled with imminent dystopia—"Nineteen eighty-four is not an inappropriate date to choose for the biological apocalypse we are facing"[3]—and he continually invokes the inevitable "suicide of the species" because of a willingness to accept this new medical technology. He seems to consider his world's relation to the future the way the Shakers conceived of millennialism: it has already begun. That is, we are already living in the end-times, and our current lives demonstrate it. Of course, for the Shakers, their ability to live in harmony was itself evidence of the arrival of the heavenly world on earth. For Ramsey, it was a looming dystopia.

Compare Ramsey's alarming description of reproductive technology to Fletcher's discussion, largely in favor, of artificial insemination. Fletcher depicts this technology not as a sign of a larger social apocalypse, but as a tool for individuals who desire children but are unable to have them. Fletcher's description lacks any grand vision of a future society; his gaze is lateral in space, not forward in time. He asks us to consider the world from the perspective of individuals who, for any number of reasons, face obstacles to having children—tragic war widows who do not want a life of "spinsterhood," a barren couple under "heavy emotional strain," and unmarried women who wish to have children. In a world populated by such sympathetic figures, artificial insemination becomes almost a "religious act"; Fletcher contends that to "transcend natural restriction, to seek ends by means devised through choice rather than by physical determinism, is a human and spiritual victory."[4] Throughout his discussion, Fletcher focuses on the manner in which technologies like artificial insemination are able to fulfill the human need for love. He stresses that parenthood is a moral, not legal, relationship with children and thus any objection based on a purely physiological basis is not "compatible with a morality that welcomes emancipation from natural necessity, or with the Christian ethic which raises morality to the level of love (a *personal* bond), above the determinism of nature and the rigidities of the law as distinguished from love."[5]

I begin this book with these two perspectives on artificial insemination, not to compare their *positions* on the technology, but to compare their *descriptions* of it: the same procedure in the same society at the same time in history. Ramsey describes artificial insemination within a frame of a society that is moving toward dystopia, akin to Huxley's *Brave New World*—that is, a dystopia we have constructed for ourselves. Fletcher describes the same technology, but within the framework of the lives of individuals whose most intimate needs are not being met because of biological barriers. Fletcher's description, in contrast to Ramsey's grand end-of-times vision, is smaller scaled: he focuses on individual humans with specific needs.

This book concerns the importance in bioethics of matters of framing, scale, and tone—essential elements of the acts of description. My central interest is the power of such choices to direct readers to see the world in a particular way. As William May has observed, ethics always entails a form of vision, but a particular type of vision of the world, for it includes within it a "corrective lens," which highlights the difference between the way the world is and the way the world should be.[6] So in bioethics, descriptions always possess within them a type of double vision, a description of how the bioethicist thinks things are, a description in the indicative mood, with an assumed counterdescription in the subjunctive mood of how the bioethicist thinks things should be. The indicative description, because it anticipates a desired agreement by the reader of the preference for a subjunctive description, is never innocent. In other words, the corrective vision corrupts the presentation of the world "as it is."

Kenneth Burke observes that

> [w]hen a writer give us a sequence of logical propositions framed to show why he got to his conclusions, he is almost reversing the actual processes of his thought. He presents data which supposedly lead to a conclusion—whereas the conclusion had led to the selection and arrangement of the data. The *demonstration* is derived from the *demonstrandum*.[7]

While the writer may have come to the conclusion first and then written the argument for that conclusion, the reader experiences the opposite; that is, the reader encounters the conclusion as a natural consequence of a series of steps. Burke's concept of form is another way to understand this relationship. Burke argued that forms of representation arouse certain desires in the reader which the writer endeavors to fulfill. His typology of this pattern included progressive form, best illustrated by a classic syllogism, and repetitive form, which can be seen in the three-part repetition of many folktales but is most notable in the structure of Western music: its repetitions, such as leitmotifs in operas, prompt the listener to anticipate the next iteration in the series—and to be disappointed if it fails to come. Conventional forms can take shape structurally, as in the metrical requirements and rhyme scheme of a sonnet, or else in the content of a work, such as a mystery's particular narrative expectations (red herrings and dead ends; the crime ultimately solved). Burke also noted the existence of minor and incidental forms.

The form of bioethics arguments also creates a desire in the reader. In bioethics, and in all applied ethics, one could argue, there is a presentation of a broken world. That presentation, in turn creates the reader's desire to learn how that world might be healed. We might think of this process as the construction of desire in descriptions of moral problems.

In an essay on the effectiveness of applied ethics in health care, Arthur Caplan notes how a "number of philosophers, theologians, and others with a major interest in ethics, have in recent times, found themselves plying their trades in the confines of a hospital or medical center," an observation that leads Caplan to ask, "are philosophers and others engaged in what has come to be called 'applied ethics' in the 'real world' of medicine able to do anything useful there?"[8] In that sentence, Caplan has two sets of quotation marks. The first set, around "applied ethics," is simply meant to indicate that this is the first time a new, technical term appears in the essay. The second, however, is a form of "scare quotes," that is, punctuation used "to alert readers that a term is used in a nonstandard . . . , ironic, or other special sense."[9] What I believe Caplan means by this second set of quotation marks is the subject of this book: that while we think of applied ethics like bioethics as applying moral reflection onto the real world, the real world does not truly exist as an entity outside of any particular perception of it. Now I am not suggesting a radical, Baudrillardian argument that the reality to which bioethics applies theory does not in any manner truly exist. What I am saying is that the world in bioethics texts is always a representation, always a creation of the author. As I will argue, each bioethics text contains within itself a particular "real world," one that should be viewed as providing rhetorical power to support and persuade us of the efficacy of a particular take on an issue—even prior to knowing what that take is. Bioethicists, whether consciously or unconsciously, construct a world for their theories and then invite us in; that world is one where theories and arguments can flourish. Ramsey and Fletcher both provide particular representations of the world through their choice of language, metaphors, historical framing, and symbolism. These choices create for the reader a coherent world that exists, and in the end supports, the argument being made.

If bioethicists create worlds in their texts, we as readers must become attuned to their constructed nature and learn to account for this in our assessment of the argument. Consider, for example, how little sense Ramsey's argument against assisted reproduction would make in the world constructed by Fletcher, or how Fletcher's yearning widows and disappointed couples have no place in Ramsey's dystopia. Both Ramsey and Fletcher are coming from the same religious tradition and generally share a notion of parenthood as an essential good. But one describes artificial insemination in terms of how it leads to the end of humanity, while the other describes it as enabling humans to fulfill their spiritual potential by transcending the limitations of biology. Bioethics prides itself on attending to the moral dimensions of the natural world, but there is nothing natural about the world that we encounter in their texts.

The power of description in academic writing is not qualitatively different from the way worlds are created in fiction. At the end of his postmodern novel *The French Lieutenant's Woman*, John Fowles openly discusses the fictionality of the novel the reader is experiencing. Fowles is a modern writer recreating the Victorian novel, so he is aware that the form does not permit "the open, the inconclusive ending." Further, while Fowles wants his characters to seem lifelike, free from obvious authorial manipulation, he is nonetheless aware that fiction is always a fixed fight. The writer of fiction places

> conflicting wants in the ring and then describes the fight—but in fact fixes the fight, letting that want he himself favors win. And we judge writers of fiction both by the skill they show in fixing the fights (in other words, in persuading us that they were not fixed) and by the kind of fighter they fix in favor of: the good one, the tragic one, the evil one, the funny one, and so on.

Fowles notes that "the chief argument for fight-fixing is to show one's readers what one thinks of the world."[10] In this novel, Fowles provides two different endings to the fight he has created. He remains aware, however, that even these apparently equal gambits cannot escape authorial partiality, as he has the power to determine the order in which these endings appear and thus can still, in essence, fix the fight.[11]

Academic arguments are no different. We are given a world in which the author has shown conflicting views, but also one where the ending, the academic's conclusion, appears natural—a necessary end to the fight. This is the power and the essence of the rhetoric of academic writing. Fletcher and Ramsey are both describing the same moral problem, but their descriptions, the power of their descriptions, is the manner in which they fix the fight. Throughout this book, we will be looking at different ways in which various bioethical fights are fixed. In short, description is a rhetorical act; when we describe the world, we tell as much about ourselves (if not more) as we do about the things being described. Richard Rorty wrote that "anything can be made to look good or bad by being redescribed."[12] In the context of bioethics, every powerful description requires a new description in order to be challenged. Major battles over key moral issues and theories in bioethics are, I contend, primarily struggles over worldviews. From this perspective, the most successful bioethicists (in terms of getting others to adopt their views) are those who are the most skilled in redescribing the world.

Take, for example, James Rachels' oft-cited argument concerning active versus passive euthanasia. In "Active and Passive Euthanasia," Rachels argues that the distinction between "assisted dying" and what is referred to in bioethics as the "withdrawal of treatment" is logically suspect. While bioethics has traditionally dissociated these two actions, Rachels argues that there is in fact little moral difference between the two. His essay is essentially a commentary on a 1973 statement that was adopted by the House of Delegates of the American Medical Association, which Rachels quotes in part here:

> The intentional termination of the life of one human being by another—mercy killing—is contrary to that for which the medical profession stands and is contrary to the policy of the American Medical Association.
>
> The cessation of the employment of extraordinary means to prolong the life of the body when there is irrefutable evidence that biological death is imminent is the decision of the patient and/or his immediate family. The advice and judgment of the physician should be freely available to the patient and/or his immediate family.[13]

Rachels next gives an example of how this illogical distinction might end up causing a patient more suffering: he asks us to imagine a "familiar type of situation" in which a patient experiences great pain while dying from cancer. If the current treatment is continued, the patient will die in a few days. But because of the pain, the patient, along with their family, asks the physician to end their life. Rachels then asks us to imagine that the physician withholds the treatment, which Rachels argues the AMA's statement permits due to the claim that "it would be wrong to prolong [the patient's] suffering needlessly." Withholding the treatment brings about the patient's death but, in doing so, prolongs the time the patient suffers. Rachels argues that once one has stopped treatment, which one knows will hasten the patient's death, they should be able to provide a lethal injection, like the withdrawal, in order to decrease the patient's suffering. So Rachels argues:

> The AMA policy statement isolates the crucial issue very well; the crucial issue is "the intentional termination of the life of one human being by another." But after identifying this issue, and forbidding "mercy killing," the statement goes on to deny that the cessation of treatment is the intentional termination of a life. This is where the mistake conies in, for what is the cessation of treatment, in these circumstances, if it is not "the intentional termination of the life of one human being by another?" Of course it is exactly that, and if it were not, there would be no point to it.[14]

In her essay "The Intentional Termination of Life," Bonnie Steinbock criticizes Rachels' argument, along with a similar argument by Michael Tooley. Steinbock's criticism focuses not on the disputed accuracy of a philosophical distinction between active and passive euthanasia, but instead on Rachels' and Tooley's interpretation of the AMA's statement. She writes:

> Whether or not the belief that there is a significant moral difference is mistaken is not my concern here. For it is far from clear that this distinction is the basis of the doctrine of the American Medical Association which Rachels attacks. And if the killing/letting die distinction is not the basis of the AMA doctrine, then arguments showing that the distinction has no moral force do not, in themselves, reveal in the doctrine's adherents either "confused thinking" or "a moral point of view unrelated to the interests of individuals."[15]

Here, Steinbock argues that Rachels, as seen in his selective quoting, is *redescribing* the AMA statement so that it seems to be drawing a simple distinction between passive and active euthanasia. Instead, Steinbock counters, the AMA is making a more subtle distinction: the cessation of the employment of extraordinary means to prolong life versus the intentional termination of life. According to Steinbock, Rachels' summary of the AMA statement, which never mentions "extraordinary means," allows him to argue for the elimination of a simple distinction that, in actuality, was never made.

What is particularly interesting in Steinbock's reading of Rachels' essay is that she shows how Rachels both gives us the text of the AMA's statement and then rewrites it in his argument to represent something different from what it says. Rachels redescribes the AMA doctrine so that it, in Rachels' interpretation, depends on an arbitrary difference between killing and letting die.

An attention to the way description persuades us of particular views even before those views are explicitly expressed fits within a tradition known as the rhetoric of inquiry. This tradition has critically examined a wide range of intellectual disciplines, from anthropology and biology to economics and jurisprudence. While rhetoric is itself a well-developed and independent discipline, advocates for the rhetoric of inquiry argue that rhetorical analysis should be an activity internal to every discipline's practice. Rhetoric is not focused primarily, as most assume, on the decoration or adornment of a core argument (a la the saying, "merely rhetorical"); it is concerned with what makes any discourse community's communications persuasive. And what many in the rhetoric of inquiry observe is that there is a sizable gap between what a discourse community *thinks* is persuasive and what actually is.

The rhetoric of inquiry looks past an imagined ideal of formal logic or rules of argumentation to analyze the way people actually make their arguments—the manner in which various disciplines are, as Herbert Simons notes, driven by "sign and analogy; by anecdotes and exemplars; and even by appeals to authority, tradition, convention, intuition, and aesthetic goodness-of-fit."[16] This concern for the way arguments are intertwined with literary devices is not to prioritize form over content or the decorative over the conceptual, but rather to attend to how those devices affect our evaluation of the argument's validity. As Diedra McCloskey, a pioneer of the rhetoric of economics, explains: "Rhetoric is not a new methodology. It is antimethodology. It points out what we actually do, what seems to persuade us and why."[17] The express purpose of the rhetoric of inquiry is to attend to the relationship of poetics to persuasiveness.

This book has a kinship with self-reflexive texts in other fields that have examined the power of description. Clifford Geertz, in *Works and Lives: The Anthropologist as Author*, looks at how ethnographic description profoundly relies upon the rhetoric of literature.

> The ability of anthropologists to get us to take what they say seriously has less to do with either a factual look or an air of conceptual elegance than it has with their capacity to convince us that what they say is a result of their having actually penetrated . . . another form of life, of having one way or another, truly "been there." And that, persuading us that this offstage miracle has occurred, is where the writing comes in.[18]

In this work, Geertz conducts close readings of the literary styles of a number of prominent anthropologists to reveal the way style persuades us of the authenticity of their accounts. In *Minding the Law*, Anthony Amsterdam and Jerome Bruner argue that legal thinking is so thoroughly entangled with the construction of stories, categories, and rhetorics that "judicial opinions, like other texts, contain the world of which they speak and, by impressing their structure on it, create it in their image."[19] Misia Landau observes that, within the field of paleoanthropology, differing explanations of human evolution feature distinct narrative variations on hero myths; she contends that laying this bare "could lead to different ways of doing science."[20] In his analysis of policy surrounding drinking and driving, Joseph Gusfield applies dramaturgical analysis to reveal the way social responses to that issue are "constructed within conventions particular to that genre of actions, just as dramas are staged with conventional understanding between audience and performers."[21] Gusfield attends to the metaphors and rituals of the construction of public policy that creates the illusion of social order.

I wish to emphasize that this book should not be read as providing a systematic method for uncovering the rhetorical elements of bioethics. I am quite catholic when it comes to theory, and I draw on a number of theorists and methods, many from fields that revolve around representation and persuasion, such as literary criticism and rhetoric, to reveal how bioethics texts work. I enlist these methods in order to do what Gusfield said Burke was doing when he created his various taxonomies and schemas: that is, "systematic thinking about the limitations of systems."[22] Each chapter spotlights a key rhetorical strategy within the discipline of bioethics, but each is only an attempt to begin to reveal the grammar of the discipline. In the end, the goal of this study parallels what Stephen Toulmin noted in his classic text on pragmatic argumentation: the work is "to raise problems, not solve them; to draw attention to a field of inquiry, rather than to survey it fully; and to provoke discussion rather than to serve as a systematic treatise."[23]

ROAD MAP

This book opens with an examination of *retrodiction*, the process by which a narrative is constructed so that it leads to a particular end. In this chapter, I will draw upon the work of the historian Hayden White, who developed a typology of various historical "emplotments." Using the template of the literary critic Northrop Frye, White argues that historians tend to construct one of four types of narrative (comic, satiric, tragic, or romantic) when they write their historical accounts. A central insight is that the end of these historical-narrative types determines the structure of the beginning. The histories created by bioethicists, usually explanations for the rise of the field starting in the 1960s, also reveal particular emplotments, and these are conditioned upon the author's vision of a possible corrective future. The new paradigm proposed, whether it be casuistry, communitarianism, virtue ethics, or a principle-based approach, drives the structure of the historical frame, so to the reader, it appears as a natural solution to the problems facing bioethics.

The second chapter examines the ways in which bioethicists employ the narrative strategy of *anagnorisis*. I take this concept from literary criticism, with its ancient roots in Aristotle's *Poetics*. Along with reversal and suffering, Aristotle saw a *moment of recognition* as a key feature of the plot. This shift, from a perspective of illusion to a sudden awakening to the truth, drives a narrative forward. In bioethics, one finds anagnorisis functioning as a rhetorical technique by which a given aspect of the world is redescribed so that we come to see the entire world as in some manner morally compromised. As May has argued, ethics should always be understood as a corrective lens. But accepting that lens requires first coming to see one's prior lens as rendering a false image of the world. In this chapter, I will look at the ways specific issues such as animal welfare, corporate influence, the Hippocratic tradition, and environmentalism are redescribed so that readers start to anticipate and desire a new vision for this fallen world.

The third chapter looks at the rhetorical power of what Burke refers to as "representative anecdotes." Burke argued that within any text, there are narrative segments that reveal the hidden grammar of a writer's motive. This chapter will engage the psychologist Jerome Bruner's take on Burke's *dramatistic pentad*—a method for assessing character motivations based on the relative weighting of five common dramatic elements—by showing how bioethicists tend to embed in their arguments short narratives that have a distinct imbalance in a specific dramaturgical ratio. This ratio allows them to subtly suggest a way to correct the imbalance.

The fourth chapter examines how what Chaim Perelman and Lucie Olbrechts-Tyteca refer to as *dissociation* functions in bioethics descriptions. In their classic work, *The New Rhetoric*, Perelman and Olbrechts-Tyteca note the manner in which arguments are made by breaking apart concepts that were initially thought of as being components of a single unity. The employment of dissociation in bioethics is so powerful because the defining and delineating of concepts is such a core aspect of the discipline. Consider concepts such as personhood, death, disability, and futility: debating and deciding their definitions is a chief role of bioethicists, and those decisions often have actual consequences in policy. To explore the nature of dissociation, I first discuss examples of "breaking the links"—arguments that do not so much establish a new division as attempt to demonstrate that we have falsely associated things that should have been kept distinct. I will then look at some examples of dissociation in bioethics: dissociating physicians from the enhancement debate, abortion from the definition of personhood, deafness from the category of disability, and sexual activity from procreation.

While dissociation is a rhetorical move that redescribes a concept so that we see a lost distinction, the fifth chapter examines persuasion through metaphor; that is, a redescription that links concepts together. While there has been a great deal of work in bioethics on metaphors within medical discourse, this chapter will look at how metaphor functions within bioethics discourse itself. One of the most notable ways is via analogical reasoning—but since this form of metaphorical thinking has already been attended to in the field, I will look at two other forms of metaphor. First, I will examine what Michael Osborn refers to as "archetypal metaphors." These are the field's central metaphors as defined by those attacking its traditional practices; identifying such archetypes becomes a way for critics of bioethics to use the metaphors by which the discipline understands itself to undermine the discipline. Second, I will discuss expressions of what Stephen Pepper has termed "root metaphors" in bioethics arguments, ultimately suggesting that disagreements in bioethics may be as much about differing root metaphors as the theoretical arguments themselves.

Chapter 6 draws upon the concept of sources of argument in the work of Richard Weaver. In an argument, Weaver submitted, one can place an emphasis on a particular source, and that source drives the description of the argument. Weaver provided a typology of various sources that can be used in the construction of an argument, which he also contended should be understood in a hierarchical structure with some sources being more ethical than others. Bioethicists also tend to draw upon a particular source for their argument, and these sources strongly influence what they focus on in their portrayal of moral problems.

Chapter 7 looks at bioethics discourse through the lens of transtextuality. Bioethics texts, like all discourse, construct a relationship between themselves and prior texts. I will examine two forms of what has been classified by Gérard Genette as "hypertextuality," the transformation of a prior text by a text or texts that come after. First, I will look at "continuation," by which bioethicists bring a prior philosophical text to bear on the field of bioethics. The second form of hypertextuality is the more interesting form for bioethics argumentation, however. This is the manner in which a bioethicist summarizes the texts of prior thinkers. While continuation is a form of extension, summarization entails a form of constriction, through which a writer re-presents a prior argument in a condensed version. This redescription will necessarily be a selection—and thus to some degree a concealment—of particular aspects of the other person's position. In order to show the rhetorical impact of summary, I will compare several summaries of one of the most influential texts in bioethics, Tom Beauchamp and James Childress' *Principles of Biomedical Ethics*. As each author summarizes this text in different ways, their "version" of the summary enables them to hide those aspects of the text that would indicate the new argument has already been anticipated in this prior text. Using summary as a form of redescription, these bioethicists create space for their text by representing the prior text as missing key features of moral arguments.

The concluding chapter looks at the concept of description and redescription in bioethics in general. I start with the importance that the notion of context has for the discipline. Next, I consider the criticism that has been leveled at what could be said to be naïve assumptions about what context *is*—or rather what it is not. Since context entails simply the combination of texts, a writer has the power to associate a moral problem with a seemingly endless number of other texts. In order to illustrate this potent form of redescription, I will look at the ways abortion has been redescribed by opponents and proponents, placing differing social texts alongside the procedure. Each "context" leads the reader to see abortion in a particular way and, in doing so, also leads to a particular moral evaluation. The ability of a bioethicist to control context is the ability to define a moral issue.

This act of representation, as well as the other types detailed in the prior chapters, is a way to persuade the reader before any particular normative position is put forth. Readers of bioethics arguments should understand the multiple forms of persuasion at work when they evaluate a text's position. Drawing on Rorty's notion that new ideas are the result of strong poets, I argue that new arguments in bioethics are primarily the result of a bioethicist's ability to show themselves to be a stronger poet than those who have come before.

NOTES

1. See J. Wesley Robb, "The Fletcher/Ramsey Debate in Bioethics and the Christian Ethical Tradition," *Religion in Life* 46, no. 1 (1977): 81–91.
2. Paul Ramsey, *Fabricated Man: The Ethics of Genetic Control* (New Haven, CT: Yale University Press, 1974), 104.
3. Ramsey, *Fabricated Man: The Ethics of Genetic Control*, 137.
4. Joseph Fletcher, *Morals and Medicine* (Boston, MA: Beacon Press, 1960), 117.
5. Fletcher, *Morals and Medicine*, 139.
6. William F. May, *The Physician's Covenant: Images of the Healer in Medical Ethics*, 2nd ed. (Lexington, KY: Westminster John Knox Press, 2000), 2
7. Kenneth Burke, *Permanence and Change: An Anatomy of Purpose*, third ed. (Berkeley, CA: University of California Press, 1984), 98
8. Arthur L. Caplan, "Can Applied Ethics be Effective in Health Care and Should it Strive to be?," *Ethics* 93, no. 2 (1983): 311.

9. *The Chicago Manual of Style* (Chicago, IL: University of Chicago Press, 2017), 435.

10. John Fowles, *The French Lieutenant's Woman* (Boston, MA: Little, Brown & Company, 1969), 417.

11. See David Lodge's discussion of Fowles' concept in David Lodge, *Working with Structuralism: Essays and Reviews on Nineteenth and Twentieth-Century Literature* (London: Routledge & Kegan Paul, 1981), 143–145.

12. Richard Rorty, *Contingency, Irony, and Solidarity* (Cambridge; New York: Cambridge University Press, 1989), 73.

13. As quoted in James Rachels, "Active and Passive Euthanasia," *New England Journal of Medicine* 292 (January 9, 1975): 78–80.

14. Rachels, "Active and Passive Euthanasia, 79."

15. Steinbock, Bonnie. "The Intentional Termination of Life." In Killing and Letting Die, edited by Bonnie Steinbock and Alastair Norcross. Englewood Cliffs, NJ: Prentice-Hall, 1980. 69–80.

16. Herbert W. Simons, *The Rhetorical Turn: Invention and Persuasion in the Conduct of Inquiry* (Chicago, IL: University of Chicago Press, 2011), 2.

17. Donald McCloskey, *The Rhetoric of Economics* (Madison, WI: University of Wisconsin Press, 1985), 51.

18. Clifford Geertz, *Works and Lives: The Anthropologist as Author* (Stanford, CA: Stanford University Press, 1988), 4–5.

19. Anthony G. Amsterdam and Jerome S. Bruner, *Minding the Law* (Cambridge, MA: Harvard University Press, 2000), 144; see also Richard K. Sherwin, "The Narrative Construction of Legal Reality," *Vermont Law Review* 18 (1993), 88–120.

20. Misia Landau, "Human Evolution as Narrative," in *Memory, Identity, Community: The Idea of Narrative in the Human Sciences* (Albany, NY: State University of New York Press,1997), 262.

21. Joseph R. Gusfield, *The Culture of Public Problems: Drinking-Driving and the Symbolic Order* (Chicago, IL: University of Chicago Press, 1981), 22.

22. Joseph R. Gusfield, "Introduction," in *On Symbols and Society*, ed. Joseph R. Gusfield (Chicago, IL: University of Chicago Press, 1989), 7.

23. Stephen Toulmin, *The Uses of Argument* (Cambridge: Cambridge University Press, 1958), 1.

Chapter 1

Retrodiction

In September of 1992, the University of Washington held a conference on "The Birth of Bioethics." Albert Jonsen, reporting on the conference, wrote that its task was to bring together some of the "pioneers" of bioethics to reflect on the discipline's history. Jonsen contends that bioethicists are only now beginning to raise such questions as: "Where did this new ethics of medicine, or bioethics, come from? What events occasioned its origins? What forms has it taken? Who elaborated it? Who pays attention to it? What is its significance for modern medicine, health care, and health policy?"[1] Jonsen, I believe, is correct that scholars had only then begun to write formal histories of bioethics. David Rothman—the first according to many—chronicled in 1991 the "most remarkable—and thoroughly controversial—transformation" in the ethics of medicine in the United States.[2] Renee Fox has written of the "evolution" of American bioethics as a "social and cultural, as well as an intellectual happening."[3] Edmund Pellegrino has described a "metamorphosis" of medical ethics from the "Quiescent Period" of the Hippocratic tradition through the Periods of Principlism and Antiprinciplism.[4] Robert Baker in *The Structure of Moral Revolutions* argues that the history of bioethics has been a series of "moral revolutions."[5]

Jonsen himself has studied the relationship between the "old ethics" and the "new medicine,"[6] and then wrote a more formal history of bioethics.[7] M. L. Tina Stevens' historical monography *Bioethics in America* takes a more critical view of the bioethics movement as the "midwife" to new biomedical research and technology.[8]

Yet, even prior to this recent self-reflective turn, speculating on the history of medical ethics in general and the bioethics movement in particular has been a familiar motif in bioethicists' arguments. Look, for instance, at the opening of Tom Beauchamp and James Childress' *Principles of Biomedical Ethics*, a work notable for its expressly ahistorical posture.

> Medical ethics enjoyed a remarkable degree of continuity from the days of Hippocrates until its long-standing traditions began to be supplanted, or at least supplemented, around the middle of the twentieth century. Scientific, technological, and social developments during that time produced rapid changes in the biological sciences and in health care. These developments challenged many prevalent conceptions of the moral obligations of health professionals and society in meeting the needs of the sick and injured. The objective of this book is to provide a framework for moral judgment and decisionmaking in the wake of these developments.[9]

Beauchamp and Childress argue that, although the writings of the past are a "rich storehouse of reflection," they are inadequate to respond to today's moral problems, and we require a new paradigm for ethics in medicine. It is a historical explanation of why the authors need not attend to history.

The passage exemplifies, however, the way that bioethicists have constructed historical narratives to explain the emergence of their discipline. This historical framing is a formal and common feature of the rhetoric of bioethics. Although Beauchamp and Childress might respond that they are simply providing the context for their arguments, understanding such "historical background" as frames allows one to remain aware that context is never simply there to be found but is itself constructed. To examine the historical framing rather than the historical contextualization of bioethics in turn allows us to see how ethicists have attempted to construct a particular concept of causality in bioethics. Implied in historical frames such as Beauchamp and Childress' is the claim that the bioethics discipline emerged not as the result of an intellectual trend in academia—like for instance cultural studies or semiotics—but rather in response to wider social changes that called for a new moral paradigm in medicine.

Not all ethicists draw upon historical frames in their arguments, but it has been a particularly prominent rhetorical strategy for those promoting a new paradigm for moral decision-making. Joseph Fletcher opens *Morals and Medicine* by tracing the prehistorical "marriage" of medicine and religion to its "divorce" in modern times.[10] Robert Veatch's *A Theory of Medical Ethics* focuses on the present uselessness of the Hippocratic tradition.[11] Richard Zaner's perspective in *Ethics and the Clinical Encounter* is intimately connected to his "historical study" of modern medicine.[12] In *Life and Death Decision Making,* Baruch Brody begins by referring to the scientific advances of the twentieth century.[13] A central feature of E. Haavi Morreim's *Balancing Act* consists of a "bit of history" that explains the rise of medicine's new economics and how this in turn affects medical ethics.[14] Revealing the rhetoric of historical frames does not expose some troublesome secret within the field but rather raises the question of whether history is being utilized in a desired and appropriate manner. Attention to the rhetoric of history permits us to look at bioethicists' arguments and "to replace simple acceptance of their reports with insightful scrutiny of their reasons."[15] The initial problem of these historical frames is that they suggest to the reader that the philosopher is responding to particular historical forces and thus the moral paradigm proposed provides the necessary resolution to the historical cause of the present ethical quandaries.

Each historical frame, I contend, must be viewed in relationship to the new moral paradigm being proposed by the ethicist. Here, someone like Rothman, a historian describing the rise of bioethics, should be distinguished from those like Beauchamp and Childress for whom the description introduces and justifies some new moral paradigm. I do not wish to suggest that Rothman is not promoting a particular way of looking at medical ethics in his history, but I think it would be difficult to demonstrate that Rothman is arguing for a particular paradigm for ethical decision-making. Beauchamp and Childress' narration not only promotes a way of perceiving the past but also a way of envisioning the future. Arthur Danto's work on the philosophy of history provides a useful framework to discuss the use of history by bioethicists. Like all historical presentations, those of bioethicists rely on a key element of historical construction, which Danto refers to as "narrative sentences." The reason this class of sentences is important for Danto is that it reflects a particular understanding of history, that is, it exposes a particular unexamined epistemological element in the philosophy of history. He explains that narrative sentences "refer to at least two time-separated events though they only describe (or only about) the earliest event to which they refer."[16] He observes that no one before 1648 would refer to the war they were in as the "Thirty Years War."[17] To illustrate this same phenomenon in bioethics writing, Jonsen advances in *The Birth of Bioethics,* "the seeds of bioethics were sown . . . during the forty years between 1947 and 1987," and the central events to which Jonsen refers are the sudden technological advances in medicine. The year 1947 for Jonsen that marks the beginning of bioethics is the year of the Nuremberg Trials, "a new beginning in the moral traditions of medicine, a beginning that would become bioethics." Stevens in *Bioethics in America* essentially attempts to rewrite this "sentence" by presenting the true beginning of bioethics can be found in the concerns "of the earliest bioethicists and 'prebioethicists'" who were "focused more acutely on the atomic bomb than on the atrocities committed by Nazi doctors on human subjects."[18] Stevens term "prebioethicsts" is an encapsulated example of Danto's point. It is difficult to imagine that anyone would ever in the present refer to them as a "prebioethicists," this is something that only takes place after there are bioethicists for which one was the embryo. For someone to identify themselves in 1945 as such would be not an act of history but rather of *prophecy*. Danto uses the term *prophecy* in reference to his analysis of narrative sentences not merely as a statement made about a particular future but a statement made by one

> who speaks about the future in a manner which is appropriate only to the past, or who speaks of the present in the light of a future treated as a *fait accompli*. A prophet treats the present in a perspective ordinarily available only to future historians, to whom present events are past, and for whom the meaning of present events is discernable.[19]

Yet as Danto observes, the condition of the narrative sentence is itself a form of prophecy, for in using such sentence structures, "they are trying to write the history of what happens *before* it has happened, and to give accounts of the past based upon accounts of the future."[20] Wallace Martin observes that in all narratives there is an intimate link between temporality and epistemology, for

> The earliest events recounted take on their meaning and act as causes only because of the later ones. Whereas most sciences involve prediction, narrative involves "retrodiction." It is the end of the temporal series—how things eventually turned out—that determines which event began it: we know it was a beginning because of the end. . . . Thus history, fiction, and biography are based on a reversal of cause-effect relations. Knowing an effect, we go back in time to find its causes.

Danto similarly notes this feature of historical narratives in that "what we select as the beginning of a narrative is determined by the end" so that a "chief task in narrative is to set the stage for the action which leads to the end, the description of which is the explanation of the change of which beginning and end are the termini."[21] Thus Paul Veyne argues that retrodiction is unavoidable in historical work, for "[h]istorical synthesis is nothing but this operation of filling in." Attending to retrodiction, this "filling in," is important to keep in mind because it permits us to see the employment of historical reflection in bioethics as a rhetorical construction. Veyne claims that historians adopt a particular plot line that in turn guides the selection of relevant material.[22] This is only one possible route the historian could take, for the stories do not exist to be found but are "found" in the plotting. Once the historian has selected a particular route, facts come forward as the material for historical investigation. Consequently, as Louis Mink has observed, there does not exist a single story to explain events but rather "there are many stories, not only different stories about different events, but even different stories about the same events."[23] But for bioethics it is not the present that determines the past, as in the historical writings analyzed by Danto, Veyne, and Martin, but rather an imagined future that determines the construction of the past. The narrative whole created is to start with an imagined ending, that is, an imagined future resolved by the moral framework envisioned by the bioethicist, and then to construct a past that leads to the present problems which can only be resolved with the new method that brings an end to bioethics. To put it in a poetically blunt way: *the purpose of bioethics theory is to bring an end to the history of bioethics*. Prophecy within this context is not so much the ability to predict the future but rather as has been shown in the phenomenology of prophets to include those that warn of potential futures if changes are not made. The introduced theory—or revival of a particular theory—is the messianic text that will resolve the reason the philosophical disease referred to as bioethics came into being. For the ethicist begins with a proposed imagined ending, a new paradigm or a solution to our present problems, and then recounts events that will lead to this imagined "closure." Since these historical frames have become such a standard part of bioethicists' rhetoric it compels us to examine critically this form of inquiry and evaluate how the arguments are used.

In *Metahistory,* White presents a "typology of historiographical styles" including forms of emplotment. By drawing upon the work of literary critic Northrop Frye, he argues that historians in their writings use four distinct mythoi or plot structures (comic, satiric, tragic, and romantic). Since these various plot structures are so much a part of how we tend to construct narratives, when creating "true" stories, we tend to draw upon these structures to frame and understand the past. White notes that he is aware that this is not the only way plottings can be classified and that a common criticism of Frye's typology is that it does not work well on the genre of the novel. Historians, however, tend to avoid complex plot structures like those of the novel and thus are "inclined to emplot" their narratives through "the most conventional forms." It is important to note that White believes that plot structure is only one of three ways that historians construct rationales for perceived change; along with ideological implication and formal argument, all three combine to form a variety of strategies that historians draw upon to create explanatory effects. For White, recognizing the choice of a particular plot structure "has its implication for the cognitive operations by which the historian seeks to 'explain' what was 'really happening' during the process of which it provides an image of its true form." White's typology of historical emplotment provides a useful framework for disclosing the way ethicists shape the history of the discipline in ways that make their philosophical approaches seem artless and self-evident; these historical reflections in turn work, like the epistemology of all narrative discourse, through retrodiction. If, as I claim, these historical forms are motivated by a need to persuade readers of the importance and validity—and in some manner the inevitability—of the moral paradigm proposed, we must re-examine historical arguments in bioethics.

THE TRAGIC HISTORY OF PLURALISM

H. Tristram Engelhardt begins *The Foundations of Bioethics* by arguing that "Contemporary bioethical questions arise against the backdrop of a fragmentation of moral perspective and vision that is closely tied to a series of losses of faith and changes in Western ethical and ontological conviction."[24] For Engelhardt, this "backdrop" includes Luther's nailing of ninety-five theses to a church door, the onset of the Thirty Years' War, the discoveries of Copernicus, and the publication of Darwin's *On the Origin of Species*. Bioethics within this historical frame is not simply the result of unique changes in the twentieth century but requires us to look to the sixteenth century for its true roots. The problems faced in bioethics are part of a breakdown in many of the suppositions of the Western worldview. Luther's actions challenged the West's belief that one could count upon "a single moral viewpoint grounded in faith, governed by a single supreme religious moral authority." The Pax Westphalica confirmed that no "one Christian vision" would bring Europe together. Copernicus' De revolutionibus orbium coelestium (1543) was one of a number of scientific discoveries "that would leave our secular vision devoid of a sense of absolute or final perspective: man ceased to be at the center of the universe." After Darwin's theory, human beings were simply another animal in the natural world. For Engelhardt, the questions raised in bioethics reflect a larger questioning of the Western Christian worldview, which began long before the arrival of dialysis or heart transplants.

The fundamental change in Engelhardt's history that has led to the bioethics movement has been the loss of a unitary moral vision. The Christian worldview that provided a "content-full" way to resolve moral dilemmas has been replaced with a secular ethic that provides no guidance for particular issues. We are left to live within a postmodern philosophical world. "The failure of the modern philosophical project to discover a canonical content-full morality constitutes the fundamental catastrophe of contemporary secular culture and frames the context of contemporary bioethics."[25]

Engelhardt plots his history of bioethics through a tragic mythos. The structure of tragedy leads downward, not toward a state of reconciliation like comedy, but toward hard-earned knowledge. In tragedy, the hero begins in a state of power but, through a quest, eventually falls and in turn moves from a state of innocence to one of experience. The denouement of the tragic plot is the resignation to the "inalterable and eternal" conditions of the world and the realization that we "cannot change them but must work within them."[26]

Engelhardt views the history of bioethics as the tragic fall of the Western Christian worldview. The West now abides in a pluralist environment, in which rationality (the driving force of the Enlightenment) cannot save us. The only thing left in the tragic plot is a resignation to the knowledge gained. The tragic tone of Engelhardt's history also appears in the preface to the first edition of his work:

> Some may wish to see this volume as a defense of a secular pluralist ethic. That would be a mistake. My intent has not been to defend that ethic but rather the very opposite. I have endeavored to find grounds for establishing by reason a particular view of the good life and securing by general rational argument the authority for its establishment. To my dismay and sorrow, such have not been available. Rather than as a manifesto on behalf of secular pluralist ethics, this volume is offered as an acknowledgment of its inevitability.[27]

In the second edition, Engelhardt clarifies his ideas concerning the tragic nature of his discovery. He contends that some have read his work as a celebration of individual freedom and thus have misunderstood his own personal convictions: "Here the reader deserves to know that I indeed experience and acknowledge the immense cleft between what secular philosophical reasoning can provide and what I know in the fullness of my own narrative to be true,"[28] for Engelhardt, himself, is a member of a particular community. He sees this book as an attempt to salvage the "wreckage of the project of establishing a secular morality that can bind all."[29] In the conclusion he once again echoes this tragic history of medical ethics by beginning with a section titled "Cosmic Disorientation."

> We find ourselves alone. We are left without ultimate purpose or orientation. We have retreated to our own devices. . . . As moral strangers, within the fabric of secular morality, we confront godlike choices with impoverished human vision, and without ultimate guideposts.[30]

This is the knowledge at the end of a tragic mythos, and Engelhardt reassures the reader that these conclusions distress him as well. He knows that there is more to the moral life than what can be discovered by reason alone, but "this is all that secular moral reasoning can provide." Given that the history of bioethics is a tragic one, in which we must acknowledge and live with the true contingent nature of the moral world, the task of bioethics is to recognize and distinguish the morality of a secular society and of a particular moral community. The secular ethic consists of those types of decisions made when several different communities, with, by definition, differing views of the Good, live together. Since rationality cannot reconcile differing ideas of the Good, only the value of toleration can be justified; only the particular communities can work out the details of what to do in individual circumstances (that is, outside the simple value of tolerance). Thus, Engelhardt argues that "Taken by itself, secular bioethics would be an empty framework," for the only principle that can be prescribed is tolerance.

Engelhardt's search for a secular ethic, which provides a necessary environment for life in a pluralistic world, fits within his historical understanding of the source of these conflicts. For Engelhardt, conflicts arise because of the fragmentation of the modern world, the breaking away through the centuries of the belief in a single worldview. This understanding of the postmodern conditions we live in determines "the limits on what may be aspired to and what may be legitimately aimed at in the quest for security and sanity in the world."[31] We do not have to respond to the moral issues of technology but, rather, to the trend toward pluralism. Engelhardt frames his argument for the development of a secular bioethics as an inescapable and tragic response to the secularization of the Western world.[32] In the end, he leaves the reader to wisdom that can only be attained by facing the unpleasant and tragic truth of the inability to achieve a unified moral vision with strangers.

THE SATIRE OF SOCIAL CHANGES

Although Albert Jonsen and Stephen Toulmin's *The Abuse of Casuistry* is conceived as dealing with a general "history of moral reasoning," the work is profoundly informed by the bioethics movement. In the prologue, Jonsen and Toulmin make an "autobiographical remark" that explains how they "came to collaborate on this 'peculiar task' of rehabilitating casuistry."[33] The authors' "shared experience" on the National Commission for the Protection of Human Subjects of Biomedical and Behavioral Research gave them insight into the "new casuistry." Although the representatives on this commission started from diverse backgrounds and justified decisions "by appealing to different 'general principles,'" they were often able to reach a consensus on cases and thereby construct a moral taxonomy. Jonsen and Toulmin conclude "the general truth and relevance of those universal principles turned out to be *less* certain than the soundness of the particular judgments for which they supposedly provided a 'deductive foundation.'"[34] The recent attention to inductive, case-based reasoning in ethics was intimately linked to the rise of bioethics as a distinct field of research.

After chronicling casuistry's birth and death, Jonsen and Toulmin trace, in chapter 16, the "revival of casuistry" in relation to a renewed interest by philosophers in moral questions in the 1960s. They see bioethics as arising in conjunction with a general concern with morality in professional fields. These challenges to authority, according to Jonsen and Toulmin, were due not so much to technological advances in medicine as to a transformation in the social climate. Although they acknowledge that the "historical reasons" for this interest in applied ethics are "complex and still partly obscure," they claim these changes had primarily to do

> with the challenges to authority and expertise that were evident in many other areas of life at this time. During the early twentieth century people in Britain and the United States had taken for granted a broad consensus about basic values. . . . During the 1960s this consensus vanished; and even professionals whose good intentions had earlier been unquestioned (first, physicians) found their integrity being called into question: So there began a discussion of issues in professional ethics—first in medicine, subsequently in business, law, and other fields—that has continued ever since.[35]

Jonsen and Toulmin conceive of the bioethics movement as one part of social changes during the sixties that took place on many levels in society, and this in turn had profound consequences for the Anglo-American philosophical tradition. In particular, this transformation came about through a challenge to conventional norms and authority. Bioethics is not a result of technological extensions but rather is the result of bringing outsiders to challenge the traditional authority of the physician. This ethos of rebellion extended not only into the professional norms of medicine but also into the norms of philosophy. "With the 1960s this older 'fact/value dichotomy' was openly challenged, and a new concreteness and particularity entered moral philosophy. So as time went on, the significance and particularity of clinical issues were better appreciated."[36]

Unlike the tragic plot structure of Engelhardt, Jonsen and Toulmin's plot is satiric: the social and philosophical worlds are turned upside down. The phrase "the new casuistry" is itself an ironic invention, for Jonsen and Toulmin, in the end, argue that we have always been doing casuistry when we apply our theories to cases. Casuistry may be abused on a meta-level, but on a more profound level, that is, the applied level, it has always been embraced by those engaged in resolving moral issues. This analysis fits the satiric mythos, which results in a "repudiation of all sophisticated conceptualizations of the world" and "anticipates a return to a mythic apprehension of the world and its processes."[37] In Jonsen and Toulmin's plot for the bioethics movement, all the previous conceptualizations are shown as inadequate, and thus an ironic unfolding occurs. While ethics had become more abstract, the realities of medicine called for philosophers to deal with the concrete moral realities. While philosophers had become more detached from day-to-day questions, they now found their ideas relevant enough for the op-ed pages of *The New York Times*.[38] While ethics concerned itself with principles, the new ethics had to respond to cases. Casuistry, once a slur, became a compliment. The Presidential Commissions demonstrated that one did not even have to talk about principles to discuss moral issues with others. For Jonsen and Toulmin, principles are tyrannical and require challenges. The historical frame that Jonsen and Toulmin construct is essentially a satiric one that connects casuistry, social protest, and the bioethics movement. Jonsen and Toulmin do not see the rise of bioethics as something that requires closure; instead, bioethics is a radical revision of moral philosophy and of philosophy's participation in society. The rise of biomedical dilemmas is not a problem to be solved but rather signifies that we are in a new and more vital time. Casuistry challenges all attempts to create lofty conceptual systems and satirically calls for a philosophy that begins in events and then moves up, rather than the other way around.

THE COMEDY OF LIBERALISM

Historical reflection, or rather historical revision, is central to Ezekiel Emanuel's *The Ends of Human Life*. In his first chapter, he attempts to challenge the view that bioethics has arisen due to advances in technology. He claims, "This view has been so widely accepted by physicians, health policy experts, lawyers, bioethicists, and the public that it has attained the status of an axiom, what we might call the technological axiom of medical ethics."[39] Emanuel's argument for a particular form of communitarianism rests on rewriting this historical narrative.

According to Emanuel, the technological axiom is based on a flawed understanding of the history of medical ethics. He admits that technological advances in medicine can "affect" issues in bioethics, but this is not the same as arguing that they have *created* these ethical issues. Issues such as confidentiality and truth-telling have been covered by the earliest moral codes formulated by the medical profession. Although technology can make these lasting issues more complex, it does not alter their essential shape. "Technology has simply outfitted these eternal questions in new clothes, but it has not altered the fundamental ethical issues beneath the new appearances."[40]

Emanuel recognizes that there does remain a central question to be addressed: "If technology has not created medical ethical issues nor their interminable irresolution, why are they on the 'public agenda'?" (Emanuel 1991, 13). Emanuel contends that the history of bioethics is, in actuality, the history of political liberalism. Bioethics thus must be seen within the context of political changes and not in terms of technological progress. Emanuel sees the rise of political liberalism not as the resolution of moral problems but as a root cause of them. "It is the failure of the political philosophy that underlies the contemporary deliberations in medical ethics, of liberalism, to provide such guidance that has created the current preoccupation with and irresolution of medical ethical questions."[41] Bioethics is not an exciting new philosophical adventure but rather a sign that all is not right with our society. Emanuel thus advocates a political solution to these problems. His argument is not for a philosophical model that will resolve these moral problems but a political framework that permits a reexamination of the communal conceptions of the Good.

Emanuel's resolution to the problems faced in medical ethics is communitarian. Medicine's ends cannot be isolated from the larger moral fabric of society. One enters into a balancing of the ends of the medical profession and the ends of the larger society. "Thus we can imagine that each profession has a sphere of its own activity, and these separate spheres are then integrated into a consistent ethical framework through political philosophy."[42] The problem with political liberalism is that it promotes no particular end. Political liberalism responds to pluralism by constructing a neutral structure in which "there should be no substantive end that is either promoted by or used to justify society's laws and policies."[43] The principle of a moral end becomes replaced in the face of "a plurality of conceptions of the meaning, purpose, and value of life" with the principle of neutrality. "On liberal grounds, the state's institutions and policies should create a political framework within which individuals who hold different views can pursue their own conception of the good life."[44] Emanuel contends that medical ethicists have attended to the wrong cause of our present problems, for they have focused on technology or decision-making rather than political philosophy. In the end, Emanuel shifts his challenge from the medical ethicists (who seem unaware of the cause and futility of their field) to the political scientists (who possess the tools necessary to resolve these problems but are unaware of the way moral issues in medicine are testing grounds for their discipline).

Emanuel's emplotment of the rise of bioethics bears a comic structure. Comic emplotments, as Frye and White conceive of them, do not so much mean periods of humor as a pattern of events that lead to a positive reconciliation.

> The reconciliations which occur at the end of Comedy are reconciliations of men with men, of men with their world and their society; the condition of society is represented as being purer, saner, and healthier as a result of the conflict among seemingly inalterably opposed elements in the world; these elements are revealed to be, in the long run, harmonizable with one another, unified, at one with themselves and the others.[45]

Emanuel's plot could have easily been tragic in the same manner as Engelhardt's if he did not envision a positive reconciliation. Both Emanuel and

Engelhardt view the rise of bioethics as a symptom of a larger problem in the fabric of society, and both see a future within particular moral communities. But their plots are substantially different. Engelhardt portrays the rise of bioethics as part of the failure of the Enlightenment project; Emanuel, as a result of a wrongheaded political structure. As Emanuel indicates, and in doing so reveals the comic mythos of his history,

> The difficulty presented by liberalism is not merely a practical impossibility arising from the multitude of views espoused in our society [as Engelhardt's work suggests]. Rather, in liberal political philosophy there is not even a theoretical way of resolving the pressing medical ethics issues.[46]

Emanuel possesses a "liberal communitarian vision of health care," a utopian vision of American society where people belong to different "community health programs" (CHPs). Each of these CHPs contains a particular conception of the Good, and Emanuel's final vision for the future of the United States is one not where "we find ourselves alone" with Engelhardt, but one in which we come to join particular communities and we find that those supposed inalterably opposed elements—communitarianism and liberalism—are "in the long run, harmonizable with one another."

THE ROMANCE OF VIRTUE

Edmund Pellegrino and David Thomasma in *The Virtues in Medical Practice* also deny the technological axiom in their historical frame: "The most crucial dilemmas of medical ethics today are not those arising from medicine's scientific progress."[47] Unlike Emanuel, however, they see this not as part of a larger shift in political philosophy but as the result of a fundamental internal dilemma within the medical profession. "In these matters, medicine faces an unenviable choice. It must reconcile two opposing orders—one based on the primacy of its covenant with patients and the other based on the ethos of self-interest."[48] Technology often brings this tension to the foreground, but it does not bring it into being. Instead, this tension has arisen because there has been a shift in the expectations of the profession. These expectations have arisen because there are social forces that seek to corrode the essential moral foundation of the medical community. Pellegrino and Thomasma argue that

> medicine is at heart a moral community . . . and . . . as a result, physicians have collective, as well as individual, moral obligations to protect the welfare of sick persons in a world that increasingly treats medicine as a commodity, a political bauble, an investment opportunity, or a bureaucrat's power play.[49]

Pellegrino and Thomasma trace the "historical antecedents" for this idea of medicine as a moral enterprise from the Hippocratic era to the eighteenth-century idea of the "gentleman doctor." They argue that this ideal has been weakened in recent years due to a series of factors.

> Specialization has divided the body of knowledge formerly held in common into dozens of pieces; medical ethics itself has focused on decision-making by individual physicians and has given little attention to their collective obligations; moral pluralism divides physicians as it does everyone else. . . . To this we must add legitimation of the profit motive, the transformation of the physician into a variety of roles—businessperson, scientist, proletarian, corporate executive.[50]

They also claim that medicine's sense of community has been distorted by a general defensive posture toward lawyers, politicians, and consumer activists. The reaction to these groups has resulted in medicine conceiving of itself as "a union, not a profession, of self-interest, not of activism."[51] While Pellegrino and Thomasma track approximately the same period of time as Jonsen and Toulmin, they do not portray the rise of the bioethics movement as a positive revision of society and philosophy, for they see medical ethics as the result of a decline in the profession due to social forces that reinforce self-interest.

Pellegrino and Thomasma's history of bioethics is fundamentally a romantic one. The emplotment of romance is an adventure in which a hero must battle clearly delineated forces of evil. As White summarizes it, the romantic plot is "a drama of the triumph of good over evil, of virtue over vice, of light over darkness, and of the ultimate transcendence of man over the world in which he was imprisoned by the Fall."[52] For Pellegrino and Thomasma, medicine is engaged in a battle against the forces of self-interest. They believe that the profession of medicine can triumph over self-interest by reinstating virtue as the foundational value. As Frye indicates, "The central form of romance is dialectical: everything is focused on a conflict between the hero and his enemy, and all the reader's values are bound up with the hero."[53] Throughout their book, Pellegrino and Thomasma set up a dialectic of the virtues of the profession versus the vice of self-interest. It is important to note that this struggle is seen by the authors as a perennial one. For instance, in their discussion of the virtue of trust, Pellegrino and Thomasma argue that this is "not a new phenomenon" but that in "the last two or three decades, these perennial sources of distrust have been reinforced and expanded."[54] Likewise the other virtues such as "justice," "fortitude," and "self-effacement" have always existed in a struggle against self-interest, but it is our recent corrupt social values that lead the profession to have to formally re-examine its moral character. Frye observed that there is a cyclical quality to the mythos of the romance, and Pellegrino and Thomasma's plot does have a similar cyclical quality. This struggle of virtue versus vice is not new; this is an ancient battle of the children of light versus the children of darkness, which each generation must take up. Because of this, Pellegrino and Thomasma's emplotment does not become tragic or comic. While Engelhardt sees his secular ethic as a realist's response to the limitations of philosophy and Emanuel envisions a reconciliation of liberalism and communitarianism, Pellegrino and Thomasma imagine the triumph of virtue over the perennial enemy of self-interest.

CONCLUSION

What is at stake in these various emplotments? To answer this question, one must once again recall the epistemological nature of narrative to be retrodictive, to see the end in the beginning because one already knows the end. I contend the battle of historical origin in bioethics is, in the final analysis, a battle over the paradigms, the proposed ends to our present moral problems. It should not strike us as odd that ethicists draw upon the emplotment that supports the paradigm they think is superior. Theory and historical emplotment become self-fulfilling prophecies. The writers would like us to believe that they are simply providing theories to help resolve the problems that arise due to particular historical causes. Consequently, histories of bioethics are driven by what the literary critic Frank Kermode refers to as "the sense of an ending."[55] Ethicists begin with an imagined ending, be it a new political structure to health care or a return to virtue, and trace a historical beginning that leads to this ending, be it one when political liberalism began or when self-interest dominated the medical culture. The historical narratives of the rise of the bioethics movement make the ethicist's paradigm appear self-evident, but we must understand this historical reflection as retrodictive rather than causal. In the final analysis, this battle over the past is a contest for the future.

Can we avoid creating plots that promote a particular worldview? One needs to remember that the critics of historical understanding, such as Veyne, White, and Mink, develop their observations on the rhetoric of history by examining the narratives of esteemed historians, not philosophers. If these critics are correct, then retrodiction is a part of the way human beings think when we reflect on the past, and therefore we will always create narratives that show the past as having a necessary causal link to some predetermined end. White rhetorically queries:

> Does the world really present itself to perception in the form of well-made stories, with central subjects, proper beginnings, middles, and ends, and a coherence that permits us to see "the end" in every beginning? Or does it present itself

> more in the forms that the annals and chronicle suggest, either as mere sequence without beginning or end or as sequences of beginnings that only terminate and never conclude?[56]

If there is anything that connects all of the histories of the discipline presented in this chapter, it is the extraordinary certitude the authors seem to possess concerning their particular "take" on the historical cause of our moral ills.

While in this chapter we have focused on the issue of time in relation to various descriptions of the historical origin of bioethics, in the next chapter we will look at the way bioethicists construct their vision of the contemporary world through a particular fusion of time and space. Like the process of retrodiction, this world-building frames the environment in which moral issues in medicine arise and contains within them a hidden cargo of an anticipated solution that exists prior to the description, which in fact guides the world being built.

In the next chapter, I will turn from larger historical-narrative frames in bioethics to the manner in which moments of epiphany are created in bioethics texts. Bioethicists often redescribe the world in a manner that reveals that we have been under an illusion, an illusion that hides a profound moral problem in the world. Just as historical frames implicitly lead a reader to view the moral world in a particular manner, through moments of what Aristotle terms *anagnorisis*, a bioethicist can create in the reader a need for a new vision of the world.

NOTES

1. Albert R. Jonsen, "The Birth of Bioethics," *Hastings Center Report* 23, no. 6 (November–December 1993): S2.
2. David J. Rothman, *Strangers at the Bedside: A History of How Law and Bioethics Transformed Medical Decision Making* (New York: Basic Books, 1991).
3. Renee Fox, "The Evolution of American Bioethics: A Sociological Perspective," in *Social Science Perspectives on Medical Ethics*, ed. George Weisz (Dordrecht; Boston, MA: Kluwer Academic Publishers, 1990).
4. Edmund D. Pellegrino, "The Metamorphosis of Medical Ethics. A 30-Year Retrospective," *Journal of the American Medical Association* 269, no. 9 (March 3, 1993).
5. Robert Baker, *The Structure of Moral Revolutions: Studies of Changes in the Morality of Abortion, Death, and the Bioethics Revolution* (Cambridge, MA: The MIT Press, 2019).
6. Albert Jonsen, *The New Medicine and the Old Ethics* (Cambridge, MA: Harvard University Press, 1992).

7. Albert R. Jonsen, *The Birth of Bioethics* (New York: Oxford University Press, 1998).

8. M. L. Tina Stevens, *Bioethics in America: Origins and Cultural Politics* (Baltimore, MD: Johns Hopkins University Press, 2000).

9. Tom L. Beauchamp, *Principles of Biomedical Ethics*, 4th ed. (New York: Oxford University Press, 1994), 3.

10. Joseph Fletcher, *Morals and Medicine* (Boston, MA: Beacon Press, 1960).

11. Robert Veatch, *Theory of Medical Ethics* (New York: Basic Books, 1981).

12. Richard M. Zaner, *Ethics and the Clinical Encounter* (Prentice Hall College Div, 1988).

13. Baruch A. Brody, *Life and Death Decision Making* (New York: Oxford University Press, 1988).

14. E. Haavi Morreim, *Balancing Act: The New Medical Ethics of Medicine's New Economics* (Washington, DC: Georgetown University Press, 1995).

15. John S. Nelson, Allan Megill, and Donald N. McCloskey, "Rhetoric of Inquiry," in *The Rhetoric of the Human Sciences: Language and Argument in Scholarship and Public Affairs*, ed. John S. Nelson, Allan Megill, and Donald N. McCloskey (Madison, WI: University of Wisconsin Press, 1991), 4.

16. Arthur C. Danto, *Narration and Knowledge* (New York: Columbia University Press, 2007), 143.

17. Danto, *Narration and Knowledge.*

18. Stevens, *Bioethics in America: Origins and Cultural Politics*, 32.

19. Danto, *Narration and Knowledge*, 9.

20. Danto, *Narration and Knowledge*, 13.

21. Arthur C. Danto, *Analytical Philosophy of History* (Cambridge: Cambridge University Press, 1965), 248.

22. Paul Veyne, *Writing History: Essay on Epistemology* (Manchester: Manchester University Press, 1984).

23. Louis Mink, "Narrative Form as a Cognitive Instrument," in *The Writing of History: Literary Form and Historical Understanding*, ed. Robert H. Canary and Henry Kozicki (Madison, WI: University of Wisconsin Press, 1978), 74.

24. H. Tristram Engelhardt, *The Foundations of Bioethics*, 2nd ed. (New York: Oxford University Press, 1996), 8.

25. Engelhardt, *The Foundations of Bioethics*, 8.

26. Hayden V. White, *Metahistory: The Historical Imagination in Nineteenth-Century Europe* (Baltimore, MD: Johns Hopkins University Press, 1973), 9.

27. Engelhardt, *The Foundations of Bioethics*, viii.

28. Engelhardt, *The Foundations of Bioethics*, xi.

29. Engelhardt, *The Foundations of Bioethics*, 8.

30. Engelhardt, *The Foundations of Bioethics*, 411.

31. White, *Metahistory: The Historical Imagination in Nineteenth-Century Europe*, 9.

32. Thomas H. Murray, "What do We Mean by Ethics and Narrative?," in *Stories and Their Limits: Narrative Approaches to Bioethics*, ed. Hilde Lindemann Nelson (New York: Routledge, 1997).

33. Albert R. Jonsen and Stephen Edelston Toulmin, *The Abuse of Casuistry: A History of Moral Reasoning* (Berkeley, CA: University of California Press, 1988), 16.

34. Jonsen and Toulmin, *The Abuse of Casuistry: A History of Moral Reasoning*, 18–19 Emphasis in original.

35. Jonsen and Toulmin, *The Abuse of Casuistry: A History of Moral Reasoning*, 304.

36. Jonsen and Toulmin, *The Abuse of Casuistry: A History of Moral Reasoning*, 305.

37. White, *Metahistory: The Historical Imagination in Nineteenth-Century Europe*, 10.

38. Stephen Toulmin, "How Medicine Saved the Life of Ethics," *Perspectives in Biology & Medicine* 25, no. 4 (1982): 736–750.

39. Ezekiel J. Emanuel, *The Ends of Human Life: Medical Ethics in a Liberal Polity* (Cambridge, MA: Harvard University Press, 1991), 9.

40. Emanuel, *The Ends of Human Life: Medical Ethics in a Liberal Polity*, 9.

41. Emanuel, *The Ends of Human Life: Medical Ethics in a Liberal Polity*, 13.

42. Emanuel, *The Ends of Human Life: Medical Ethics in a Liberal Polity*, 26.

43. Emanuel, *The Ends of Human Life: Medical Ethics in a Liberal Polity*, 33.

44. Emanuel, *The Ends of Human Life: Medical Ethics in a Liberal Polity*, 35.

45. White, *Metahistory: The Historical Imagination in Nineteenth-Century Europe*, 9.

46. Emanuel, *The Ends of Human Life: Medical Ethics in a Liberal Polity*, 33.

47. Edmund D. Pellegrino and David C. Thomasma, *The Virtues in Medical Practice* (New York: Oxford University Press, 1993), 31.

48. Pellegrino and Thomasma, *The Virtues in Medical Practice*, 32.

49. Pellegrino and Thomasma, *The Virtues in Medical Practice*, 32.

50. Pellegrino and Thomasma, *The Virtues in Medical Practice*, 34–35.

51. Pellegrino and Thomasma, *The Virtues in Medical Practice*, 35.

52. White, *Metahistory: The Historical Imagination in Nineteenth-Century Europe*, 9.

53. Northrop Frye, *Anatomy of Criticism: Four Essays* (Princeton, NJ: Princeton University Press, 1957), 187.

54. Pellegrino and Thomasma, *The Virtues in Medical Practice*.

55. Frank Kermode, *The Sense of an Ending: Studies in the Theory of Fiction* (New York: Oxford University Press, 1967).

56. Hayden V. White, *The Content of the Form: Narrative Discourse and Historical Representation* (Baltimore, MD: Johns Hopkins University Press, 1987), 24.

Chapter 2

Anagnorisis

Peter Singer, one of the most influential philosophers of the late twentieth century, has worked on many issues, including justice and clinical ethics. He is best known, however, for his challenges to "speciesism." Speciesism is a term Richard Ryder originated for the belief that there is a qualitative and moral difference between humans and other animals. For Singer, speciesism is the reason humans are able to justify their instrumental approach to other species: it sanctions the use of animals for such things as food, clothing, and medical experimentation. Singer's preeminence on this issue has led some to call him the founder of the animal rights movement. Such a claim is simultaneously correct and incorrect. It is correct because Singer's 1975 *Animal Liberation* has been widely read not only outside philosophy but outside academia entirely, and it is certainly responsible for stimulating broader public attunement to animal suffering. Yet it is incorrect to refer to Singer as the founder of the animal *rights* movement, for to use the language of "rights" is in many ways counter to Singer's philosophical perspective as a thorough utilitarian. It is only through his utilitarian lens that Singer comes to the conclusion that speciesism is immoral; he never suggests that animals hold fundamental inalienable rights. This nuance becomes clear when we contrast Singer's philosophical perspective to that of someone like Tom Regan, who has explicitly argued against speciesism on the basis of rights. Regan is quite clear that he finds utilitarianism inadequate in providing a full enough moral theory to respond to speciesism.[1] So we are left with a puzzle. If the arguments in *Animal Liberation* were not what prompted so many people to stand against speciesism, why is the book such a key text in the movement? How does Singer persuade readers to reject speciesism if not by way of the *reasons* he offers for rejecting it?

Ramona Ilea, in an essay titled "Singer, Wittgenstein, and Morally Motivating Examples," tries to resolve this puzzle by downplaying Singer's philosophical perspective in favor of his writerly descriptions. As Ilea observes, most philosophers attend primarily to the first chapter of Singer's book, the chapter in which he lays out his utilitarian argument. By attending almost solely to this chapter, most philosophers, according to Ilea, view *Animal Liberation* as putting forth a relatively conventional utilitarian argument for how humans should view other animals. Ilea notes, however, that the book is "unusually structured," for half of it "is filled with examples and descriptions: emotionally powerful, detailed, rich, and unusually ordered."[2] Drawing on Wittgenstein, Ilea systematically analyzes this half of the book, where Singer supplies numerous vivid examples of the mistreatment of animals, from scientific research settings to the conditions on farms. Ilea's analysis is persuasive and explains why non-philosophers have been so influenced by Singer's work—without in any manner adopting his theory.

Ilea's analysis of Singer reveals a common rhetorical move in bioethics, which I will refer to as *anagnorisis*. I borrow this word from literary criticism, where it is normally translated as "recognition." The term has its origin in Aristotle's *Poetics*, in which anagnorisis (ἀναγνώρισις), along with reversal (περιπέτεια; peripeteia) and suffering (πάθος), is one of the central components of plot. Anagnorisis is the moment in which something that has been hidden from a character is finally revealed; the revelation precipitates what Aristotle calls "a change from ignorance to knowledge."[3] Aristotle thought that the best type of these moments also entailed a reversal, and cites as the classic example the moment in Sophocles' *Oedipus* where Oedipus recognizes who he is—a recognition that, in turn, causes a dramatic reversal in the plot for Oedipus. Anagnorisis can also be seen in Euripides' *The Bacchae*, in which Agave, driven to ecstasy by the god Dionysus, helps murder her son Pentheus and then proudly returns home with his head in her arms, thinking she has slain a mountain lion. Cadmus, her father, finally forces Agave to recognize that the head she carries is not a mountain lion's, but that of her own son.

While Aristotle derived the concept from ancient Greek texts, instances of anagnorisis can be found throughout literature. Take Charles Dickens' *Great Expectations*, with its famous scene when Pip's benefactor reveals himself, totally unexpectedly, to be the convict Magwitch. There is also the moment in the novel *Fight Club* when the main character discovers that his violent anarchist friend Tyler Durden is simply a part of his own psyche. These examples of anagnorisis (and Oedipus') are of a personal nature, of course. Their revelations concern personal identity, first and foremost, even when they drive the plot in a new direction. In this chapter, I wish to discuss a different type of anagnorisis, one more relevant to the poetics of bioethics: what we might call "global anagnorisis."

Found most often in speculative fiction, global anagnorisis is the moment when the world as it has been seen is revealed to be false. Unlike the moment of personal anagnorisis, this is a revelation about the very nature of the society or reality the character inhabits. To be more precise, it is a recognition that the individuals in the story have lived with a false understanding of their world. Roz Kaveney links such narratives to the philosophical concern of "cognitive dissonance," and sees the trope playing out most often in science fiction when "a world of consensual reality . . . breaks down under examination and proves to be a delusion and most usually a snare created to keep the reason prisoner."[4] In the film *Dark City*, for example, the protagonist John Murdoch comes to realize that he is not in a real city but rather in an alien-constructed environment that has been set up to create experiments to understand humans. Perhaps the most cited example of global anagnorisis is in the film *The Matrix*, in which the main character is actually given the choice to see the world as it truly is (a computer construct streamed into his brain), or to continue living in the simulation in ignorance. There is even a moment when one of the characters agrees to betray the other humans so that he can essentially reverse his own anagnorisis and return to not knowing.

The world envisioned in *The Matrix* has often been compared to Descartes' thought experiment in *Meditations on First Philosophy*, where either a deceiving God or an evil demon provides us with a world that we experience as real but is in fact an illusion. A more contemporary version of this premise is put forth by the philosopher Gilbert Harman in his 1973 work *Thought*. Instead of an evil demon, Harman proposes as the master manipulator the figure of a brain surgeon: someone who, in making patients believe the world is a particular way, is ultimately leading them to experience a world that is not authentic. The progenitor of this theme in Western literature is Plato's "Allegory of the Cave," found in Book VII of *Republic*. The allegory starts with a number of prisoners chained their whole lives inside a cave; all they know of the world are the shadow images projected by men who place objects in front of a fire. The prisoners believe that what they see, the shadows on the cave's wall, are the real world. Socrates asks his audience to then imagine if one of the prisoners were released from his chains and dragged out of the cave to see the actual real world. The man, Socrates suggests, would be confused, pained, and even resentful of this moment of illumination. Socrates ends his account by contemplating how the man would be treated once he returned to the cave with his new knowledge. He would be taken for a madman, Socrates concludes, and might even be considered dangerous enough to be killed. *The Matrix* is in many ways an elaboration of this story. The film cleverly envisions a future after the development of general Artificial Intelligence in the twenty-first century that results in a war between humans and this new intelligence. Humans create a nuclear winter to blot out the sun and take away the machines' access to power. Instead of shutting down, however, the machines capture and sedate humans, converting the bodies into their new source of energy. To keep the humans content, the machines construct a "matrix," a virtual world in which humans "live," inert, while their energy is being harvested. Neo, the main protagonist, believes he is in the late twentieth century (the time period used in the matrix), but in actuality it is the end of the twenty-second. All of this is revealed to Neo after he makes the decision to take the "red pill," which will awaken him to the real world, rather than the "blue pill," which would allow him to remain in the simulation. It is Neo's choice of the red pill that leads to the moment of anagnorisis in the film.

In science fiction, the most common revelation is not simply that the world is different than we think it is, but that it is much, much worse. (Neo is far from the only sci-fi protagonist to learn that he has been living in a dystopia all along.) Yet I would include in the category of global anagnorisis less shocking instances of insight as well. For example, in Lois Lowry's young adult novel *The Giver*, the protagonist learns that his society, which exists without want, does not in fact contain an "Elsewhere" for those in the society who are not considered desirable; those individuals are actually killed. Unlike *The Matrix*, this protagonist is not provided with a revelation of the false nature of his understanding of reality itself, but with his understanding of his social world, a world that he has been up until now deceived into believing is beneficent toward all. It is this type of "recognition"—being shown what the world is truly like and having the world before unmasked as an illusion—that constitutes the rhetorical form of anagnorisis found in bioethics arguments.

Let us return now to Singer's book *Animal Liberation*. In chapter three, "Down on the Factory Farm . . ." Singer opens by noting that for most humans, "especially those in modern urban and suburban communities," the most common form of contact made with other animals is when we eat. That is, we encounter animals as we eat them. As Singer describes,

> Buying food in a store or restaurant is the culmination of a long process, of which all but the end product is delicately screened from our eyes. We buy our meat and poultry in neat plastic packages. It hardly bleeds. There is no reason to associate this package with a living, breathing, walking, suffering animal. The very words we use conceal its origins: we eat beef, not bull, steer, or cow, and pork, not pig. . . . By using the more general "meat" we avoid facing the fact that what we are eating is really flesh.[5]

Singer continues his redescription by acknowledging those who remain aware of what they are eating, even when the product—meat, poultry—does not resemble its source. Digging into the nature of that awareness, however, he finds the "top layer of a much deeper ignorance of the origin of our food."[6] They may understand that their food comes from a farm, for instance. But as Singer points out, when they think of a farm, they imagine "a house; a barn; a flock of hens; a herd of cows being brought in from the fields for milking, and perhaps a sow rooting around in the orchard with a litter of squealing piglets running excitedly behind her."[7] The rest of the chapter is Singer's deconstruction of this tableau. It is here, Ilea argues, that the powerful rhetorical aspect of Singer's work lies:

> Singer tries to get us to see what hens are like and what the production of eggs in factory farms actually involves by providing us with numerous examples and vivid descriptions of battery cages and common practices, such as debeaking.[8]

Rather than the philosophical application of utilitarianism, then, Singer's powerful descriptions of abuse—a series of examples that counter prevailing illusions about modern farms—are the true source of his persuasiveness. They also fit the definition of global anagnorisis: Singer begins by making manifest our image of a farm before administering the red pill of reality, forcing us to see the falseness of that image. The effect of anagnorisis, when done by such a powerful writer as Singer, is that once the illusion is broken, we cannot return to our previous ignorance. The "we" here, it should be noted, is different than it is in drama and fiction; the experience of recognition is felt not by a character within a story but by the reader of Singer's work. In his historical study of the interpretation and application of anagnorisis, Terence Cave observes that this "transference of recognition from character to reader and spectator is a modern development."[9] David Lodge elaborates,

> [i]n the retelling of a well-known story like that of Oedipus, the surprise is experienced by the characters rather than the audience, for whom the primary effect is one of irony. . . . The novel, however, differs from all previous narrative forms in undertaking . . . to tell wholly new stories.[10]

For bioethics texts, of course, the notion that anagnorisis resides in the reader's experience makes sense, because, unlike novels, bioethics descriptions are accounts of our world. Often the key to anagnorisis as a rhetorical move is the exposure of some unseen moral wrong, an illusion that the author replaces with a description of how things truly are. The following examples of global anagnorisis in bioethics will demonstrate how common this rhetorical move is, and, I believe, how effective.

RECOGNIZING THE ENVIRONMENTAL CRISIS IN THE HOSPITAL

Jessica Pierce and Andrew Jameton begin their book, *The Ethics of Environmentally Responsible Health Care,* by discussing how environmental factors affect human health. They detail how dramatic changes in the global environment have led to a lack of clean drinking water and sanitation for at least half of the world's population—the cause of death for seven percent of the human population each year, they report—and note that chemical agents are central factors in the increased number of illnesses worldwide. They also observe, however, that mainstream bioethics has in recent years started to acknowledge the profound impact a devastated environment can have on health. Their subsequent summary of how health and the environment are intertwined, while undeniably important, is not exactly new information for the field. The environment may not yet be at the center of bioethics discourse, but many bioethicists have argued that it should be. To me, Pierce and Jameton's true focus does not begin until the fourth chapter, "Environmental Aspects of Health Care," for it is in this chapter that they shift their attention from the ways in which health is affected by the environment to the way health care affects the environment.

The authors begin the chapter by describing a series of prints by the artist Karl Bodemer that can be found in the halls of one of Nebraska Health System's hospitals. (Both authors were on the faculty of the University of Nebraska Medical Center during most of the book's research and writing.) The artworks are of the Nebraska prairies in the nineteenth century and include images of Native Americans and elk. Pierce and Jameton note the startling difference between these images of the Nebraska landscape and the "white coats, industrial glass and tile, and sharp fluorescent lights" of the medical center that now exists in that same space. It is at this point that Pierce and Jameton begin their redescription of the hospital, not as a place of healing but as itself a source of illness. The central argument of their book is that the hospital does not simply respond to those harmed by the environment; in many ways, it contributes to the very environmental disasters causing those harms. They support this argument by detailing the hospital's massive resource consumption as well as its production of waste, both in terms of used medical supplies and hazardous materials. "The delivery of health care in an industrialized society has complex and far-reaching ecological reverberations," they write.

> Industrialized health care in the developed nations requires large quantities of fossil fuels, plastics, medicinal plants, electricity, water, chemicals, minerals, paper, and concrete. The production, distribution, use, and disposal of

> health-care-related materials composes a portion of the overall ecological burden of all nations, especially of those in the First World.[11]

Rarely do the authors mention the reason all of this toxicity is generated—that is, to help heal and care for the sick. In their description, the word *hospital* could easily be replaced with the word *factory*; indeed, when the authors discuss medical research, they use the term "industrial health care." One of the key features of their argument is this attempt to create global anagnorisis around the role and function of the hospital. In Pierce and Jameton's redescription, the hospital is transformed from a place of healing to a vector of illness.

In the chapter that follows, the authors present their vision for an alternative to the current medical environment. They call this alternative the "Green Health Center," or GHC. The majority of this chapter is a commentary on a working group at the University of Nebraska Medical Center tasked with developing—or "envisioning," as they put it—a hypothetical GHC. Their use of the word "envisioned" reveals an important aspect of global anagnorisis, especially in the context of ethics. After all, as William May explains in *The Physician's Covenant*, *vision* enjoys a special prominence in Western philosophy and theology. Taking the allegory of the cave as one example, May notes that Plato relied on the metaphor of vision to chart "the movement from ignorance to knowledge" and connect this movement "to the painful ascent from the darkness . . . into the blinding glare of the sun."[12] May goes on, however, to discuss how ethical vision is different from the vision we get from science, in that ethics strives to also provide a "corrective lens"—what he describes as "a knowledgeable revision of the world that human practice presents."[13] Once the act of anagnorisis occurs, the ethicist now has the opportunity to envision the way the world should be. The GHC is Pierce and Jameton's revision of the environmental dystopia of the medical environment; it is their utopian replacement. Most moments of anagnorisis in bioethics are accompanied by such a revision, a future triumph over the reality that they have exposed.

THE HIPPOCRATIC CULT

Robert Veatch's *A Theory of Medical Ethics* aims to resolve various moral issues in bioethics through a contractual ethics model. Before Veatch argues for this approach, he characterizes all prior work in the field as "a series of unsystematic, unreflective, ethical stances or traditions."[14] In other words, no *theory* of bioethics can really be said to exist. Veatch argues that what is needed is a "systematic structuring" which can provide health-care professionals, policymakers, and the rest of us a way of knowing our moral positions in relation to those of people with whom we disagree. Veatch, however, must first counter any responses to this position of the lack of any universal moral foundation to medicine, and he recognizes that one source that many may cite for such a foundation (at least for Western society) is the Hippocratic tradition. Veatch makes an arresting set of claims regarding the Hippocratic tradition.

> Physicians should be able to grasp that if they opt for the Hippocratic formula . . . they are standing in a peculiar, and very particularistic tradition. It is one that at times is compatible with, but at its root is alien to, the ethics central to our culture.[15]

It is at this point that Veatch draws on a form of anagnorisis in his redescription of the Hippocratic tradition. While many medical schools in the United States still use a modern version of the well-known Oath, suggesting its status as broadly applicable even in contemporary health care, the reader is made to see that the oath is instead the expression of the values and worldview of a singular, secluded community.

This anagnorisis occurs primarily in Veatch's first chapter, "The Hippocratic Tradition." The chapter opens with an ethics case where a physician is confronted with a dying mother who wishes assistance in killing her child, to "spare her the inevitable misery of her existence" after the mother's death.[16] After presenting the case, Veatch argues that the first task is to distinguish "medical ethics" from "physician ethics." The former concerns the application of moral theory to issues in medicine, regardless of who faces the particular problem. Physician ethics concerns itself instead with the moral issues that fall solely within the sphere of physicians. For the mother in this case, observes Veatch, the perspectives given within the sphere of the various medical professions provide little assistance in resolving her moral dilemma; professional codes developed to respond to physician ethics have the potential to determine only what the physician should do. Veatch looks to the Hippocratic tradition to see if it can provide guidance on how to resolve this moral dilemma, for he points out that this tradition, especially as it is embodied in the Hippocratic Oath, is "the single most often-cited summary of the physician's own understanding of what is morally required to be a good medical doctor."[17] Veatch bluntly argues that if that tradition *cannot* provide the mother with a way to resolve her moral dilemma about killing her daughter, then a system of ethics that provides universal guidance in medicine must be found outside of that particular tradition.

One of the central arguments in this chapter, and the monograph in general, is that the profession's moral tradition has been profoundly shaped by its origin in the Hippocratic corpus of ancient Greece. Zeroing in on the Hippocratic Oath, Veatch notes that it has two distinct parts. First, there is a pledge of allegiance to the physicians who are the trainee's teachers; second, there is the promise to follow what Veatch calls "some rather strange rules of medical ethics and etiquette."[18] For Veatch, the Oath's pledge of allegiance—as well as its vow of secrecy—"is patently offensive to the modern rational mind."[19] Veatch turns to the scholarship of Ludwig Edelstein for the historical context behind such priorities. Where the loyalty feature of the Oath had been considered by others to indicate a tradition of adoption of the student by the teacher, Edelstein states that there is little evidence to support this claim. As Veatch notes, however, Edelstein found evidence that pedagogical adoption *was* practiced in that same period by the Pythagoreans. Veatch describes the Pythagoreans in the following manner:

> Pythagoras, like Hippocrates, was an Ionian Greek who gave rise to a society—a cult, if you like—with religious, political, and philosophical interests. It elevated pursuit of knowledge to the level of a religious quest. The knowledge, viewed as cultic, was protected by bonds of secrecy.[20]

Veatch's characterization of the Pythagoreans as a "cult" (if you like) is vital to his argument. By categorizing them as such and by reinforcing the relation of Pythagoras to the Hippocratic tradition ("like Hippocrates . . ."), Veatch is subtly redescribing the Hippocratic tradition as a "cult." (This terminology is particularly resonant considering that Veatch was writing during a time when the word "cult" had become entangled with a moral panic over people being "brainwashed" by various groups, ceding control over their lives, and becoming lost to society.) Veatch's argument against the use of the Hippocratic ethic as a universal code for medicine can be seen in his central anagnorisis, through which Veatch reveals "how bizarre and controversial this Hippocratic ethic is and how strange it would be if modern, rational people, whether operating out of religious or secular moral frameworks, were to revive the ethics of the Pythagorean-Hippocratic cult."[21] As Veatch has it, the Hippocratic code is not an expression of universal values, but "a minority document for an isolated group of physicians."[22]

Let us compare this characterization to other descriptions of the Hippocratic tradition in bioethics. Look, for example, at the way Grant Gillett depicts the tradition in *Bioethics in the Clinic: Hippocratic Reflections*. Gillett's second chapter, titled "Hippocrates' Children," explores the essential ideals of this tradition and argues why they should form the ethical core of contemporary medicine. The following summarizes his view:

> The Hippocratic corpus envisages knowledgeable professionals, who consult their colleagues, are free from envy and avarice, and form an honorable company dedicated to relieving suffering and a respect for persons. They have, from time to time, to make decisions involving considerable risk of harm, and sometimes they proceed urgently in the face of uncertainty under the necessity imposed by mortal danger. These are the realities of clinical practice, which cannot be regulated as if it were based on the certainties beloved of scientists and accountants, and which relies on the sound intuitions and wise judgments that are the stuff of virtuous conduct informed by extensive clinical experience.[23]

Gillett tends most often to refer to Hippocratic practitioners as a "school"; his reference to them here as "colleagues" and "professionals" contrasts markedly with Veatch's cult members, as well as his characterization of them as paragons of virtue. Or take, for example the description of the Hippocratic tradition in Leon Kass' *Toward a More Natural Science*. In this text, Kass praises the Hippocratic Oath as being a model for contemporary medicine because it has "a profound understanding of what medicine is and must essentially be."[24] As Kass sees it, the Oath "stands as *an* expression of the medical ethics *in which the medical and ethical are as hard to separate as the concave and the convex*."[25] In contrast to Veatch, Kass views the Hippocratic Oath as an expression of the essential nature of medicine, which he views as profoundly entangled with morality. We may also consider the preface to Joseph Fletcher's *Humanhood: Essays in Biomedical Ethics* (published just three years prior to Veatch's), in which he places contemporary medicine in relation to classical Greece. Fletcher writes that during the classical Greek period, the practice of medicine "was done according to the Dogmatist cults as exemplified by Empedocles and Pythagoras; it was based on metaphysics and religion. Under the leadership of Hippocrates, they broke away and based their medicine on empirical rather than metaphysical foundations."[26] Contra Veatch, Fletcher here draws a stark line between the "cults" and Hippocrates' progressive, empirical medical practice. And May, in his argument for a morality of medicine grounded in a notion of the physician's covenant, reinforces that view of the Hippocratic tradition, insisting on its direct connection to current AMA codes.[27] For these writers, Hippocrates represents a key turning point in medical practice, toward epistemological and moral progress. Contemporary medicine, in their minds, should not only continue to see the Hippocratic tradition as its hereditary foundation but should also embrace it for the future of medicine.

Veatch attempts to overturn both the understanding of the past and the basis for the future contained in these positive depictions. His subsequent chapters move away from this Greek "cult" to survey different medical ethics across the world. He begins by describing the "dominant Western competitors" to the Hippocratic tradition, focusing first on the Judeo-Christian tradition as a contrast to what he refers to as the "modern secular West." Veatch then looks at medical ethical theories outside of the "Anglo-American West," including the traditions of Islam and Hinduism and those found in China, Japan, and what was then the Soviet Union. This structure—opening with the redescription of the Hippocratic tradition, then embarking on a whirlwind survey of the ethics of the world—contributes to Veatch's larger aim of creating a new foundation for bioethics, one that is not reliant upon any particular tradition.

In Veatch's text, there are two instances of anagnorisis: one is the redescription of the Hippocratic tradition as an isolated cult, and the second is a radical decentering of any universal claim that medicine has a particular internal morality. For Veatch, sweeping away the false notion of some inherent universal ethic gives communities the freedom to create a new ethics that can reflect and bear out their particular moral values. It is those broader moral agreements that form the primary social contract to which the medical profession must conform. This is the first part of Veatch's notion of a "triple contract," which entails a basic social contract, a contract between society and a profession, and a contract between particular professionals and particular patients. Throughout his discussion of the "triple contract," Veatch returns to attack the Hippocratic tradition as a core impediment to its realization. When describing the limited value of the principle of beneficence, for example, Veatch spends a sizable portion of his criticism detailing how problematic the concept is in the Hippocratic tradition. And when he discusses the "second principle of the social contract," he goes so far as to say that the Hippocratic tradition "is totally devoid of any notion of promises made to outsiders."[28]

Veatch's presentation of the Hippocratic tradition as radically other and isolated from the contemporary world of medicine is a motivated critique. It is meant to show that there is no tradition to which contemporary practices owe a debt, no need to justify modern ethics with respect to this prior tradition. By refuting this living lineage, Veatch is able to create a blank slate for the creation of a new ethic. Lacking any history allows the freedom to create an ethic that need not respond to a prior history of practice.

THE FOUNDATIONS OF PATRIARCHAL BIOETHICS

> Ours is a world permeated by sexism. In virtually every sphere of life, women's interests are systematically subordinated to those of men; and yet, these arrangements are so extensive, so familiar, and so entrenched in our habits of thought that it is possible not to notice them at all.[29]

This is the opening passage of Susan Sherwin's *No Longer Patient: Feminist Ethics and Health Care*. In many ways, this attempt to make evident the manner in which we no longer notice the way our society oppresses women in all aspects of life is the central thesis of Sherwin's monograph; the book could be described as one extensive anagnorisis of the sexism that lies under the surface of medical ethics—and also in the discipline of bioethics.

One of the most powerful rhetorical features of *No Longer Patient* is the sustained redescription of bioethics as unable to perceive the sexism that influences every aspect of medical care. Sherwin is explicit that she is not attempting to provide a global revision of bioethical concerns, although she does remark that "[f]urther surprises and insights would ensue if other familiar bioethics topics [allocation of resources, mental illness, the right-to-die] were addressed from the perspective of feminist ethics."[30] But Sherwin does apply a feminist lens to several of the field's central issues, including abortion, reproductive technology, paternalism, and research ethics. She also explores areas she thinks a feminist perspective could usefully pull into the field of bioethics, such as the pathologizing of women's lives and the way society attempts to control women's sexuality. What is most potent about Sherwin's work is the manner in which she sees bioethics not as a source of liberation but as a discipline that ignores—and even supports—women's oppression.

> Even though medical ethics is meant to be critical of all morally unacceptable medical practices, it has failed to oppose those that contribute to the oppression of women. By not opposing them, it has implicitly supported patriarchal policies within [the?] medical establishment.[31]

Underneath the arguments made by bioethicists, regardless of where they stand on particular positions, Sherwin uncovers implicit biases making them unable to see that their decisions exist within a system of power that harms women.

Throughout the book, Sherwin presents an issue, contrasts how medicine and bioethics view the issue, then shows how both of these views leave the major features of oppression in place. In her discussion of new reproductive technologies, for instance, Sherwin notes how bioethics has traditionally viewed such questions through the concept of autonomy: asking, that is, whether an informed person can, without coercion make a free choice to use this technology. In essence, traditional bioethics has "solved" the issues surrounding reproductive technology through the frame of "the consumer freedom to purchase technology."[32] As Sherwin counters, however, this solution hides the manner in which these "reproductive technologies threaten to reinforce the lack of autonomy that most women now experience in our culture—even though these technologies appear to increase particular aspects of freedom for some women."[33] Viewing the ethics of reproductive technology as simply an issue of individual choice hides the larger social forces that compel women to bear children, even if doing so puts their own lives at risk, and so bioethics does not attend to the implicit sexist bias within IVF. Similarly, she points out, non-feminist analyses of the moral issues surrounding abortion focus on the morality of the act, which has utterly occluded the morality of variable *access* to those services. For Sherwin, framing abortion as an individual choice ignores the political features subtending the debate—and thus acquiesces to a broader system of oppression.

In her discussion of research ethics, Sherwin critiques another favored bioethical "solution," in this case the reliance on informed consent to prevent the potential exploitation of research participants. This focus on individual consent cannot come close to addressing larger moral issues of women as vulnerable subjects in research on human subjects, who are just a vulnerable population as prisoners and children.

> Medical manipulation has made women a readily available population for research by guaranteeing their disproportionate presence in medical institutions. The monopoly that medical practitioners have achieved over the management of all phases of normal female development has provided researchers with an easily accessible population of healthy subjects for use in nontherapeutic research. . . . As an oppressed population, women are likely to be considered relatively expendable, making them likely candidates for expose to risks form which more valued members of society would be protected.[34]

Here once again, Sherwin shows that bioethicists have been unable to see how their focus on informed consent blinds them to the hidden oppression that continues even within such oversight. Any moral assessment of research must be done "in terms of its connection with existing patterns of oppression and domination in society," Sherwin concludes.[35]

The rhetorical power of Sherwin's work resides in this ongoing subversion, this unveiling of how bioethics not only responds inadequately to moral problems but in many ways perpetuates them, specifically those subjugating women and other oppressed groups. Traditional bioethics becomes an oblivious collaborator of oppression rather than the guardian against oppression. Ultimately, my definition of global anagnorisis aligns with a key benefit of a feminist perspective, as described by Sherwin: to demonstrate

> that the greatest danger of oppression lies where bias is so pervasive as to be invisible. Hence, it is necessary to ask questions about all sorts of practices that have heretofore been accepted as normal. Within the fields of both medicine and bioethics, feminism reveals that we need to make conscious efforts to consider

what ethical questions may be hidden from view in our ordinary assumptions about health care.[36]

CORRUPTION OF THE MEDICAL PROFESSION

Both the title and cover of Carl Elliott's *White Coat, Black Hat* reflect the central rhetorical move of the book: the redescription of contemporary medicine as a profoundly compromised enterprise. The cover, which depicts a man in a clinical white coat wearing a black cowboy hat, is an image of clashing icons. The white coat is a nod to the medical profession's own representational ploy of adopting a lab coat as uniform in order to portray contemporary medicine as a "science." The black hat recalls the shorthand in American iconography of the white hat as the good guys and black hats as the bad guys. The fact that the black hat on Elliott's cover is a cowboy hat reinforces this echo of the American myth of the "Wild West," which was always a play between good and evil. In his oft-cited structuralist study of the Western genre, *Sixguns & Society*, Will Wright breaks down the genre's characters into three central categories: an outsider hero, a villain who is both a part of and apart from society, and the weak townspeople. The villain's role is quite complex in that he is someone well-versed in society while being fundamentally opposed to its values. The driving force of this difference is typically grounded in capitalist greed. The good guys, the ones wearing the white hats, are outsiders who come into a town whose community's values have been perverted.

In the classic Western, Wright observes, these values revolve around how and why people acquire wealth—a trope that Elliott cannily repurposes to apply to modern medicine. As Wright explains, it is not that the good people in a Western are poor and the bad ones are rich, but that each has different reasons for acquiring capital. The white hats want to use wealth to build community; the black hats acquire wealth only for their self-interest.[37] In Elliott's redescription of American medicine, the ones wearing white have become as corrupted as the greedy capitalists. This revisionist western is one in which medicine has lost its moral vision because it has joined with the black hats of Big Pharma and for-profit health care. In Elliott's Western plot, we discover that not one person is in fact wearing a white hat.

Each chapter of Elliott's book redescribes an aspect of contemporary medical practice—the compensation of human research subjects, the credibility of academic publication, the prescribing practices of physicians—where the central moral principles of medicine have been debased by a relationship with corporations, which by their telos are focused on the acquisition of capital. In his discussion of current research practices, he overturns the traditional image of research subjects as volunteers whose participation in clinical trials stems from altruism. The *Handbook for IRBs* draws a bright line between providing funds to research participants as a "reimbursement" versus as an "inducement"; it is this second category, the authors agree, that creates several morally problematic issues.[38] Here Elliott details the rise of the "professional guinea pig": individuals, often on the margins of society, who have made becoming test subjects for stage one drug trials a form of employment. These are not altruistic figures choosing to sacrifice for the common good; they are "employees" of the research enterprise. Elliott finds a similar arc applying to academics. Research publications have traditionally been vectors for the free exchange of ideas by experts who receive no direct reimbursement for the time they spend writing and reviewing articles. Yet as Elliott shows, there now exists an entire profession of individuals who act as ghostwriters for academics. The medical industry both pays for the ghostwriting and secures the academics' willingness to be listed as authors for articles that support the company's products. Further, Elliott notes, the journals themselves rely financially on the pharmaceutical industry's advertisement buys and purchased reprints of the articles used to market their products, so now not only are its articles but the journal itself funded by industry. Next, Elliott redescribes the practice of evidence-based medicine. Physicians are expected to make decisions about medical care based solely on evidence, and to always put the health of their patients first. Yet drug reps from the pharmaceutical industry have profoundly influenced the prescribing patterns of individual physicians, Elliott reports, and some of those physicians have been groomed by pharmaceutical companies as "thought leaders" in order to influence their peers on what drugs are best for patients. In the end, Elliott turns his eye to bioethicists themselves—people who have often thought of their work not only as an academic field but also as a form of social activism. Elliott presents these would-be activists as coopted by the biomedical industry, their activities funded through a close relationship with the industry itself. Elliott sees bioethics as often financially dependent upon the biomedical industry for the support of centers and the salaries of its faculties.

Throughout his book, Elliott takes traditional understandings of medicine and bioethics and provides a powerful form of anagnorisis by redescribing them as corrupted by the biomedical industry. Just as Sherwin uncovers all aspects of medical practice (including bioethics) as revealing hidden gender oppression, Elliott redescribes all of contemporary medical practice as morally compromised—including bioethics. I want to be clear that I am not in any manner arguing that these redescriptions are in some way flawed: that hospitals are beacons of environmental conservation, for example, or that capitalism has not affected medical practice. What I am doing is demonstrating one aspect of how bioethics makes arguments.

CONCLUSION: THE RHETORIC OF THE HIDDEN DYSTOPIA

Like the film *The Matrix*, the red pill that these bioethicists offer is one that reveals a dystopian world. Medicine does not heal; it is itself a source of illness. The Hippocratic tradition is not an expression of universal moral values but a religious cult. Bioethics does not liberate people by promoting health but is itself a part of patriarchal oppression. Medicine may have once had an altruistic core, but it is now a lackey of contemporary capitalism.

The darkness of these visions makes sense when we recall what May identified as the job of ethics: *revision*. Revision requires that one must first be persuaded that the world is in some fundamental way in need of it. As this chapter has shown, one way this has been accomplished in bioethics is through global anagnorisis, a trope associated most with the science fiction genre. Anagnorisis is simply one part of the plot of bioethics, for it essentially prepares the reader for what Aristotle refers to as peripeteia, the reversal of a narrative's direction. Anagnorisis and peripeteia are often viewed as linked together, in which the revelation, as in *Oedipus*, in turn leads to a reversal of the plot's direction. In bioethics, the anagnorisis should lead the reader to anticipate an alternative theory that will provide the hoped-for denouement of the plot, that is, an end to whatever has been revealed in the bioethicists' redescription—be it speciesism, anti-environmentalism, universalism, sexism, or corrupted altruism.

While global anagnorisis entails the revelation of a grand false narrative, bioethics as a discipline is also dominated by smaller narratives that function rhetorically. In the next chapter, we will turn to the use of what Kenneth Burke refers to as "representative anecdotes." These small narratives often encapsulate an entire argument. Bioethicists use representative anecdotes to reveal an imbalance in the medical world that their theory will attempt to correct. As in anagnorisis, the use of representative anecdotes in bioethics is a way to describe the world as in some manner broken and requiring a new vision, a new narration.

NOTES

1. See Tom Regan, *The Case for Animal Rights*, Updated with a new pref. ed. (Berkeley, CA: University of California Press, 2004), 349–351.

2. Ramona Ilea, "Singer, Wittgenstein, and Morally Motivating Examples," *Between the Species* 22, no. 1 (2017): 3.

3. Aristotle, *The Complete Works of Aristotle: The Revised Oxford Translation. Vol. 2*, ed. Jonathan Barnes (Princeton, NJ: Princeton University Press, 1984), 1452a.

4. Roz Kaveney, *From Alien to The Matrix: Reading Science Fiction Film* (London: I.B. Tauris, 2005), 64.

5. Peter Singer, *Animal Liberation: The Definitive Classic of the Animal Movement*, Updated ed. (New York: Ecco, 2009), 95–96.

6. Singer, *Animal Liberation: The Definitive Classic of the Animal Movement*, 96.

7. Singer, *Animal Liberation: The Definitive Classic of the Animal Movement*, 96.

8. Ilea, "Singer, Wittgenstein, and Morally Motivating Examples," 5.

9. Terence Cave, *Recognitions: A Study in Poetics* (Oxford: Clarendon Press, 1988), 260.

10. David Lodge, *The Art of Fiction: Illustrated From Classic and Modern Texts* (New York: Viking, 1993), 71.

11. Jessica Pierce and Andrew Jameton, *The Ethics of Environmentally Responsible Health Care* (New York: Oxford University Press, 2004), 44.

12. William F. May, *The Physician's Covenant: Images of the Healer in Medical Ethics*, 2nd ed. (Lexington, KY: Westminster John Knox Press, 2000), 1.

13. May, *The Physician's Covenant: Images of the Healer in Medical Ethics*, 3.

14. Robert Veatch, *Theory of Medical Ethics* (Basic Books, 1981), 5.

15. Veatch, *Theory of Medical Ethics*, 5.

16. Veatch, *Theory of Medical Ethics*, 15–16.

17. Veatch, *Theory of Medical Ethics*, 20, 18–19.

18. Veatch, *Theory of Medical Ethics*, 20.

19. Veatch, *Theory of Medical Ethics*, 20.

20. Veatch, *Theory of Medical Ethics*, 21.

21. Veatch, *Theory of Medical Ethics*, 23.

22. Veatch, *Theory of Medical Ethics*, 23.

23. Grant Gillett, *Bioethics in the Clinic: Hippocratic Reflections* (Baltimore, MD: Johns Hopkins University Press, 2004), 39.

24. Leon Kass, *Toward a More Natural Science: Biology and Human Affairs* (New York: Free Press, 1985), 228.

25. Kass, *Toward a More Natural Science: Biology and Human Affairs*, 228. Emphasis in the original.

26. Joseph F. Fletcher, *Humanhood: Essays in Biomedical Ethics* (Buffalo, NY: Prometheus Books, 1979), 5.

27. William May, "Code, Covenant, Contract, or Philanthropy," *Hastings Center Report* 5 (December 1975): 29.

28. Veatch, *Theory of Medical Ethics*, 184.

29. Susan Sherwin, *No Longer Patient: Feminist Ethics and Health Care* (Philadelphia, PA: Temple University Press, 1992), 13.

30. Sherwin, *No Longer Patient: Feminist Ethics and Health Care*, 8–9.

31. Sherwin, *No Longer Patient: Feminist Ethics and Health Care*, 88.

32. Sherwin, *No Longer Patient: Feminist Ethics and Health Care*, 134.

33. Sherwin, *No Longer Patient: Feminist Ethics and Health Care*, 134.

34. Sherwin, *No Longer Patient: Feminist Ethics and Health Care*, 162.

35. Sherwin, *No Longer Patient: Feminist Ethics and Health Care*, 134, 174–175.

36. Sherwin, *No Longer Patient: Feminist Ethics and Health Care*, 10.

37. Will Wright, *Six Guns and Society: A Structural Study of the Western* (Berkeley, CA: University of California Press, 2008), 140.

38. Robert J. Amdur and Elizabeth A. Bankert, *Institutional Review Board: Member Handbook* (Burlington, MA: Jones & Bartlett Learning, 2022), 120.

Chapter 3

Trouble

In the previous chapter, I examined the way bioethicists use anagnorisis as a rhetorical move that reveals an incorrect vision of the world. One of the texts I examined was Carl Elliott's *White Coat, Black Hat*, in which Elliott shows how capitalism has entered almost every area of American health care, corrupting its altruistic telos. Yet Elliott does not begin his monograph with a moment of anagnorisis or with an illustration of this corruption, but instead with a curious anecdote from his brother Hal's residency in psychiatry. During the residency, one of Hal's colleagues was a recent MD from Harvard who also had a PhD in neuroscience. While this resident was highly valued by the faculty, Hal always felt there was something odd about him. Eventually, the resident was exposed as a fraud. He had not attended medical school, did not have a degree in neuroscience, and may never even have graduated from college. Still, he was able to fool the people who interviewed him for the residency, and had been able to give the impression to the faculty that he was an outstanding candidate. Since this person disappeared after being exposed, Elliott is not able to share what his motivation was. One could speculate that it was for financial gain. Or perhaps the man was a pathological liar, motivated by the pleasure of the deception itself—like a medical Frank Abagnale, the conman made famous by the film *Catch Me If You Can*. Unlike the descriptions in *White Coat, Black Hat* of how the profit motive has perverted scientific research, academic medicine, and the prescription of pharmaceuticals, however, this story of personal fraud does not seem directly relevant to the book's central thesis, for, while fascinating, there is no indication that this resident was in any way illustrative of the various corruptions of medicine that are the focus of Elliott's argument. The connection Elliott himself provides is that the resident's ability to deceive is akin to the many incidents of fakery Elliott has come to see throughout contemporary medicine.

This story acts in Elliott's monograph as what Kenneth Burke terms a "representative anecdote." For Burke, certain stories can function as synchronic representations of discourse, a small part of the text that expresses the essence of the text as a whole; the representative anecdote becomes a "lens, filter, or template through which the critic studies and reconstructs the discourse."[1] These anecdotes are typically textual segments excerpted from the discourse itself, but sometimes critics will construct their own representative anecdote, which they believe acts as a synchronic encapsulation of the text.[2] As Burke conceived it, the ultimate goal of the representative anecdote was to serve as an object for a *dramatist analysis*, an investigation that uncovers a writer's motives, or, to use the often-cited beginning of Burke's *Grammar of Motives*, "What is involved, when we say what people are doing and why they are doing it."[3] Burke's notion of a dramatistic perspective comprises five elements, which he terms the dramatistic "pentad": agent, act, purpose, agency, and scene. There has been some debate in relation to Burke's comments that he wanted to add "attitude" to this grouping.[4]

In responding to some questions concerning the pentad, Burke noted that his selection of terms echoes a passage in Aristotle's *Nicomachean Ethics*: "A man may be ignorant of who he is, what he is doing, what or whom he is acting on, and also what instrument he is doing it with and to what end . . . how he is doing it . . . ."[5] Burke goes on to annotate Aristotle's "how he is doing it" as "(e.g., whether gently or violently)—which would indicate why I would class 'how' (*quomodo*) with 'attitude.'"[6] Yet his driving interest is not to thoroughly define each term but to draw attention to their interaction; as he puts it, "my stress is less upon the terms themselves than upon what I would call the 'ratios' among the terms."[7] One should not examine the pentadic terms in isolation but instead in relation to one another, so when given a description we should look at each of the various pairings such as act/scene, purpose/agency, and agent/act. Burke contended that in a description, the writer will in some manner favor one of the terms over the others, so that one of the terms will affect the character of the other terms. Take, for example a description of suicide. Psychologists like Alex May and David Klonsky describe suicide with a lens that gives dominance to the agent;[8] descriptions by philosophers such as Glen Graber[9] or Margaret Battin[10] tend to stress purpose over the other terms; and sociologists, such as Emile Durkheim, emphasize how the scene influences all the other elements of the pentad.[11] A dramatist analysis has been applied to a variety of descriptions, including Edward Kennedy's explanation of the Chappaquiddick incident,[12] public discourse over gay rights,[13] the argument over the status of midwifery,[14] and bioethicists' analysis of the cause of medical mistakes.[15] In all these cases, pentadic analysis constitutes a "strategic method for analyzing discourse by focusing on how it attributes motivation to human action."[16]

The psychologist Jerome Bruner has acknowledged the influence of Burke's pentadic model on his understanding of the narrative mode of the human mind, asserting that a crucial element of what he refers to as "story stuff" borrows from the interplay of Burke's terms.[17] But Bruner's understanding of pentadic ratios is quite different from Burke's (and almost all rhetoricians who characterize their analysis as an application of Burke). For Bruner, the pentad allows us to see what causes the drama of a narrative. This cause is always, for Bruner, the result of a particular imbalance in the pentad, which he terms the narrative's "Trouble."[18] Bruner explains that Trouble arises

> when an Act toward a Goal is inappropriate in a particular Scene, as with Don Quixote's antic maneuvers in search of chivalric ends; when an Agent does not fit the Scene, as with K in Kafka's *The Trial* or with Nora at home in Ibsen's *A Doll s House*; or when an Agent's Goal seems hopelessly unattainable given the Means available, as in Jamaica Kincaid's touching *Annie John*.[19]

It is questionable whether all narrative can be understood in terms of Bruner's notion of Trouble, for many narrative theorists view narrative as representing an *event* or *happening* which, depending on one's definition of these concepts, may result from an imbalance—or may not.[20] (A narrative could be a representation of change totally unrelated to an imbalance.) Exploring the difference between Bruner's use of ratios and Burke's, Matthew Althouse and Floyd Anderson note that while Bruner always credits Burke for his understanding of Trouble, there is no place in Burke's *Grammar*—or in any of his written works—where "Trouble with (or without) a capital T" can be located.[21] In order to resolve this mystery, Althouse and Anderson corresponded with Bruner and discovered that Bruner's understanding of how to use the ratios actually came from a number of casual conversations he had with Burke.

It could be argued that the difference between Bruner's and Burke's understanding of the ratios is a matter of focus: Bruner's is on the *fabula* of the story (the basic story material), while Burke attends more closely to the *sjužet* (the particular arrangement of the story by a particular teller). Bruner's interest is indicated by the section of *Troubled Minds, Possible Worlds* where he injects his concept of Trouble into his discussion of fabula.[22] Burke, on the other hand, is interested in the manner in which the same elements of the fabula are presented according to different motives. Althouse and Anderson conclude that Bruner's understanding of Trouble is most probably more Bruner than Burke. Yet they also argue that Bruner's use of Burke's pentad and ratios provides a new method for rhetorical analysis; one can use Bruner's concept of Trouble to investigate "how violations of cultural norms, and the ensuing complications of Trouble, may be charted."[23]

To return to the representative anecdote in *White Coat, Black Hat*, the basic pentad could be described as a conman (agent) for personal gain (purpose) acting as a physician (act) in a hospital (scene) by fabricating information (agency). While some may feel that the trouble in Elliott's description resides in an imbalance within the scene of a health-care system based on capitalism, I think a stronger argument is that the imbalance resides in a mismatch between agent and act. Once the trouble of the anecdote is characterized in this way, one sees it as an encapsulation of Elliott's entire argument. Each of the moments of anagnorisis in the book are those in which the wrong agents are doing the acts. Non-researchers doing research; professional guinea pigs acting as "voluntary" subjects in research studies, pharmaceutical companies designating who is an expert, bioethicists performing public relations. Perceiving the misaligned ratio in Elliott's argument leads to another insight: that the rhetoric of misalignment invites the expectation of a particular realignment. Implicit in a bioethics narrative of an imbalance is an appropriate response to that imbalance. For Elliott, the cause of the American health system's imbalance is the commercialization of medicine, which has created corrupt agents performing the acts of health care. Eliminating the use of medicine as a means for financial benefit and reintroducing principled agents would restore the balance.

In what follows, I will look at a number of representative anecdotes in bioethics texts; in each example, we will see that the bioethicist describes a specific ratio imbalance as the source of the problem that needs to be resolved. To put Bruner and Burke's language together, one could describe these anecdotes as "representative trouble." Typically appearing at the outset of the text, these narratives not only portray a particular imbalance, but also contain the pathway back to balance—the root of the bioethicist's argument. In some manner, there are always two representative anecdotes in bioethics. There is a narrative of imbalance and also an implied prior narrative of balance, the social conventions that existed prior to the violation. The representative anecdotes in bioethics could themselves be seen as existing within a narrative that moves from the exposure of a violation to the realization of realignment and a return to balance.

Representative anecdotes in bioethics are not simply examples of ethics cases. The key difference between the two is narratological: unlike the ethics case genre, representative anecdotes tend to be integrated into the progression of the general argument; their implied author is the same as the book's. Case narratives, on the other hand, are usually set apart from the main text and presented as if they were written by someone else. In other words, they appear to be quotations from another person (even when they are written by the author). This distinction is not universal, however. In his essay "The Case Study as Representative Anecdote," John Cash argues that case studies act as representative anecdotes for many academics.[24] Bioethics texts tend to be filled with case studies, though, so when a particular case study is also a representative anecdote, it usually falls outside the normal series of cases presented for analysis. A good example of this can be found in the third edition of Al Jonsen, Mark Siegler, and William Winslade's *Clinical Ethics*. Unlike the prior two editions of their pocket guide for clinicians, the third edition includes a more extensive introduction to their method of presenting and analyzing issues in terms of four categories: medical indications, patient preferences, quality of life, and contextual features.[25] Their book is filled with cases, each clearly presented and separated from the rest of their "comments" and "counsel." This new introduction provides a more detailed (and markedly less generic) presentation of the Dax Cowart narrative. Cowart in the 1970s suffered an accident in which he was severely burned. Throughout his treatment, Cowart requested that treatment be stopped, but the physicians caring for him felt they had a moral duty to continue to provide treatment. The Cowart case becomes a representative anecdote of Jonsen, Siegler, and Winslade's method. Unlike all the other case presentations, the narrative is integrated and told within the categories rather than simply told in relation to a particular category. Their analysis of the Cowart case through the four categories allows them to demonstrate that their method actually brings in detailed elements that are not present in the initial presentation, elements that are often missing in a pure medical presentation, which only focuses on medical indications. It illustrates the manner in which one needs to attend to all four of these categories in order to "make a case."[26]

Ethics cases become representative anecdotes when they encapsulate what, for the bioethicist is the emblematic imbalance in medicine. The argument following the presentation of such cases is meant as an explication of how this imbalance can be resolved. It is for this reason that bioethicists will often return to this representative case in the conclusion of their text; such cases are used to frame the argument overall. Representative anecdotes can be understood as a form of *paradiegesis*, a term from classical rhetoric meaning a vivid story used to introduce an argument.

EMANUEL'S IMBALANCE OF AGENCY-PURPOSE

In the prior chapter on the construction of historical retrodiction, we examined the plotting of Ezekiel Emanuel's *The Ends of Human Life*. Though it is his central focus, Emanuel does not begin with a historical explanation of how "medical ethical *questions* have become irresolvable medical ethics *dilemmas*."[27] Instead, he begins with a story of a patient, whom he introduces in a Melvillesque way: "Call him Andrew." Andrew suffers from AIDS as well as numerous other illnesses related to the syndrome. At the moment, he is in the ICU, semiconscious but unable to communicate. The question facing Andrew's physician, Dr. Wolf, is how best to care for him at this time, especially considering the conflicting requests from Andrew's partner and Andrew's family. Emanuel sees the decision as one that involves the physician-patient relationship, appropriate medical interventions, and the allocation of resources. After citing these larger categories at play, Emanuel provides a long list of relevant ethical questions. Concerning the issue of what medical interventions to employ, for example, Emanuel asks:

> Is death better than Andrew's existence on a respirator? Is Andrew's situation "a miserable death"? What future does Andrew have anyway, even if he survives? Is there "no reasonable expectation" of his recovering a meaningful quality-of-life? Was there such an expectation during the previous admission? Should he be DNR even if the respirator is not withdrawn? Should the hospital ethics committee be consulted? What is the best care for Andrew?[28]

Emanuel relates this story not because it is out of the ordinary, but because it isn't. It is simply another example of the "endless irresolution" of the moral dilemmas in contemporary medical care.[29] And we are mistaken if we think that technology is the cause of these dilemmas, according to Emanuel. Technology, such as the interventions that are now possible for Andrew, does not pose a novel moral problem; it merely puts a new face on the same problems health care has struggled with for decades. Emanuel places such issues among Thomas Nagel's category of "mortal questions," those matters that are interconnected with "the eternal human experiences of death, parenthood, personal identity, justice, freedom."[30] The problem is that we lack any agreed-upon moral framework for resolving mortal problems *in general*, not just deciding to apply this or that intervention.

The ratio that is in tension in Emanuel's representative anecdote is that of agency to purpose. Contemporary medicine does not lack possible actions or interventions. What we lack, Emanuel argues, is knowing what the final purpose of the act should be. In Emanuel's view, this problem is larger than medicine. Liberal democracy, because of its focus on process, does not provide any distinct notion of what the goals of life are. It provides the fiction of a purpose in promoting individual rights—but those rights have no content if they are not connected to some prior idea of the good life. Lacking communal agreement on this essential definition makes no one decision any better than another. Even with a great number of potential acts, not knowing their purpose, their final telos, means that we do not know how to decide on what action to take. We must first know what the purpose of health care is before we know the particular choices we should make in relation to specific medical interventions. One can only, for Emanuel, decide that purpose within a community.

In the book's concluding chapter, Emanuel returns to his representative anecdote. He states that any attempt to decide on a course of action by applying a liberal political concept of rights will be "futile," for appeals to rights "are merely procedure; by themselves they do not indicate what substantive ethical decisions should be made."[31] Emanuel does suggest "positive advice," which is essentially to reprioritize the elements of Burke's ratio and place purpose before agency. It is only in embracing a communitarian bioethics—only in seeing the problems facing bioethics in relation to a community's understanding of the ends of human life—that one can even begin to find satisfactory decisions about what actions are appropriate. Otherwise, we are left only with the "illusion of resolution" that a focus on process provides. By acknowledging the imbalance illustrated in Emanuel's representative anecdote, we can begin to revise bioethics in a manner that actually brings an end to currently irresolvable moral questions. As with Dr. Wolf and Andrew, we too must start first with a vision of the purpose of human life. The irony of this presentation of imbalance is that Emanuel is unable to provide any particular balance to the specific situation that Andrew is in, for the purpose, the vision of the good life, can only come from a particular community, not from any particular individual. The corrective narrative can only be told by a deliberative process that encompasses not merely the context of the hospital but society in general. Furthermore, Emanuel does not believe that physicians should wait for others to provide a particular vision of the good life, but instead should be a part of the process of deliberation.

HALPERN'S IMBALANCE OF AGENCY-ATTITUDE

Jodi Halpern begins her book *From Detached Concern to Empathy* with "The case of Ms. G," a narrative evaluating a woman's ability to refuse life-saving treatment. The fifty-six-year-old Ms. G had recently had her second above-the-knee amputation, Halpern recounts, and while she was a candidate for a transplant because of kidney failure, she refused the dialysis needed to keep her alive until a kidney was available. As a psychiatric resident, Halpern was charged with determining the patient's decision-making capability. Halpern learns that Ms. G's husband had told her that because of the amputations, he no longer found her attractive and had found a new partner. When Halpern raises this context to the supervising psychiatrist, he acknowledges her findings and agrees that it may explain Ms. G's refusal of treatment. Still, he says,

> The decision is hers. She has the capacity to decide, even though she's very upset. Anyway, if we set aside our own emotional reactions, especially our wishes to rescue, it is an objective fact that she faces a terrible future. We need to leave this woman to die in peace and guard against imposing our own wishes on her.[32]

After a conference with the various team members caring for her, the decision is made to respect Ms. G's wish to refuse treatment, and she dies.

Both the form of deliberation and the patient's outcome are central to Halpern's overall argument. As a representative anecdote, it condenses the critique she has toward medical practice (and in some ways toward bioethics as well).

> The medical team, ethicist, and the supervising psychiatrist sought to respond in a professional way to Ms. G's suffering. To avoid judging her situation in an emotional manner, they tried to focus on what they assumed to be objective facts, as if ticking off items on a checklist: Was she cognitively impaired? Did she have the legal right to refuse treatment? Had attempts been made to establish a therapeutic alliance?[33]

For Halpern, the key problem in the handling of this woman's case was its attitude of detachment. Physicians have been taught to practice detached concern when attending to the needs of patients; responding in this manner is justified on the grounds that it supports objectivity, which allows a physician to attend to the reality of the clinical situation. In this way, the physician is encouraged to adopt the lens of a scientist looking at an object rather than a subject caring for another subject.

The imbalance in Halpern's narrative is between agency and attitude. In the story of Ms. G's evaluation, the scene of the hospital is correct, the agents involved are correct, and the agency of engaging Ms. G in conversation and getting her point of view is correct. What is misaligned is the attitude toward the act of determining her capacity, which profoundly imbalances the purpose of the act itself. For Halpern, the purpose of the encounter should be to heal the patient. The attitude of detached concern eclipses this purpose, training the focus instead on the physician's comportment. In this imbalanced version of medicine, going through a series of set questions to determine if Ms. G can make decisions is all that is required; without the aim of healing, the application of the checklist is completely inappropriate care.

At her book's close, Halpern returns to the story of Ms. G, this time to suggest a way to restore the balance of healing-focused care. Once detached concern is replaced with an attitude of empathy, she explains, the purpose of the engagement shifts as well.

> The visual metaphor of the "objective" doctor standing before the patient and "seeing through" her irrational emotions ought to be replaced with a paradigm in which the patient "makes use of" the doctor's nonretaliatory emotional presence to go through the necessarily irrational emotional phases of grieving. This model would make it possible to transform how doctors respond to patients like Ms. G, whose certainty that her future was hopeless should trigger reflection and empathy.[34]

This narrative correction—the essential act of reimagining the representative anecdote through a new lens—conveys in Halpern's book an implicit criticism of bioethics. Ms. G's case is not an ethics case hinging on whether a patient has the right to refuse treatment, but a medical case of healing a patient in pain. The narrative is retold when the imbalance is corrected so that the purpose is transformed by the appropriate attitude toward the patient's situation.

LINDEMANN'S IMBALANCE OF AGENT-ACT

Hilde Lindemann opens her book *Narrative Identities, Narrative Repair* with a story of a group of nurses planning a Nurse Recognition Day that occurs annually at a hospital in a small Midwest city. Like other representative anecdotes in bioethics arguments, Lindemann returns to this one throughout the book as she constructs a larger argument about ethics, identity, and narrative. The point-of-view character in the anecdote is Virginia Martin, who has volunteered to be a part of the steering committee. The diverse group of (women) nurses organizing the yearly event engages in extended discussions about the qualities that an "admirable nurse" possesses. Instead of sticking with the intrinsic qualities of nurses, however, the discussion turns to what these professionals are up against—the problems they have encountered during the course of their own nursing work. One of the nurses shares a story about caring for a sixteen-year-old boy with leukemia who was not told that he was dying. The nurse caring for the boy felt he could handle the truth—that there was no cure—but when she expressed her opinion to the boy's oncologist, "he was abrupt, telling her that she was emotionally overinvolved and professionally out of line."[35] Over a series of meetings, the nurses relate numerous personal narratives in which their professional identity was not respected by physicians.

The common imbalance in these narratives is between agent and act. The nurses were continually being told that they were the wrong agents to be taking on particular acts. While this judgment was partly based on professional hierarchy, Lindemann shows that it was also because the nurses were perceived to be acting out emotional, rather than rational, responses. An orthopedic surgeon discounts one nurse's opinion that a medical consult is needed for a patient with high blood pressure. A nurse is reprimanded by the night-shift supervisor for not following a physician's orders to place restraints on a disoriented elderly patient. "Bit by bit, the nurses connected one fragment of their story to another, offering ethical interpretations of the various anecdotes and telling fresh ones that, in the light of these interpretations, now seemed relevant."[36] In each case, the nurses are not viewed as professionals with the status to decide on and carry out actions, but instead as non-agents who must follow orders without consultation.

What is unique about Lindemann's representative anecdote is that it is a representative anecdote about representative anecdotes. Each of the nurses tells a story that reveals the lack of respect they receive in the medical setting, stories in which they are told that they are not the correct agents, even when their intended actions turn out to be more informed and skillful than the ones they were ordered to perform. What these stories communicate, then, are false narratives, false imbalances: if they omitted the interpretative gloss of the disapproving physicians, they would simply recount various nurses performing actions that helped their patients. There would be no trouble. The tension in Lindemann's text resides *after* the nurses propose or take action, when the judgment of others calls those actions into question. Notably, that questioning is not whether the patients benefited from the action, but whether the nurse had the authority to suggest it. Lindemann's representative anecdote is one in which nurses come to see that their narratives are only worth narrating to the degree they are being misread as stories of imbalance: that is, when they are deemed to be inappropriate agents of appropriate acts.

This insight about storytelling is central to Lindemann's argument about the importance of narrative construction to personal identity formation, and in particular, the way false narratives or master narratives can harm one's identity. One of the reasons that Lindemann's representative anecdote contains such a strong point-of-view character in Virginia Martin is that it ends with Lindemann's desired correction, that of narrative repair. As Lindemann describes,

> The stories ultimately contributed just as much to her [Martin's] change of heart as the people who told them. . . . They spoke to her own experience, but because they were the other people's stories, the stories of people she was fond of, they aroused feelings of indignation that her own experiences had never seemed to merit. And since they were *her* stories as well, the patterns they displayed of contempt for women had to be acknowledged as a pattern in her own life. That acknowledgment made it possible for her to agree that the doctors' story about nurses, as the others were piecing it together, needed to be resisted.[37]

Lindemann's representative anecdote is remarkable both for the way it diagnoses a false imbalance as the problem and for the way it foregrounds truer narratives as the solution. In the act of exposing the false imbalance asserted by doctors, nurses like Martin are able to construct a *counterstory* of competence, marginalization, and eventual solidarity.

In her concluding chapter, Lindemann once again returns to this representative anecdote, highlighting the liberatory practice of correcting the record. After undergoing their narrative-driven "change of heart," she writes, "The committee members [now] judge their actions according to the evaluative standards of their chosen community—standards less morally defective than those used by the moral mainstream."[38]

RENÉE FOX AND JUDITH SWAZEY'S IMBALANCE OF AGENCY-SCENE

Renée Fox and Judith Swazey's essay "Medical Morality Is Not Bioethics—Medical Ethics in China and the United States" concerns Fox and Swazey's six-week stay in a Chinese hospital. They note early in the article that their title is "a rather mischievous one," for it refers to an earlier article published in the *Hastings Center Report* by H. Tristram Engelhardt. In that essay, Engelhardt recounts his own stay in China, which lasted two weeks. Fox and Swazey's retelling of Engelhardt's exploration of the state of bioethics in China is an essential intertext for their own exploration. They compare Engelhardt's travels to those of the Christian missionaries in the sixteenth and seventeenth centuries who came to conclude that the Chinese lacked "logic." They criticize Engelhardt for perceiving the moral perspective of Chinese professionals as an expression only of Communist philosophy, without recognizing how those views also connect to Confucian, Taoist, and Buddhist philosophies, each with its own long history in Chinese thought. They note that Engelhardt was unable to understand the "resistance" of the Chinese thinkers he spoke with—their unwillingness to ground their moral opinions with what he would consider a systematic philosophy. The story of Engelhardt's blindness to "the pattern and logic of today's Chinese thought," write Fox and Swazey, "is related to inadvertent ethnocentricity of the implicit premises on which his article rests. Bioethics, particularly its philosophical aspects, is viewed as largely *a*cultural and *trans*cultural in nature."[39] In Fox and Swazey's essay, Engelhardt's failure to understand the roots of morality and medicine in China acts as a representative anecdote of the failure of American bioethics to attend to social and cultural context.

So why do Fox and Swazey believe that four additional weeks allowed them to appreciate Chinese medical morality in a way that Engelhardt was unable to do in two? The difference, it turns out, is less about time and more about method. After quoting Engelhardt's characterization of his article as a "traveler's report" of his time in China, Fox and Swazey describe theirs as a "medical sociological journey" to perform a "mini-ethnography." The difference here is one of expertise as well as orientation: Engelhardt only possesses the intellectual equipment of a trained philosopher, while the authors bring the skills of sociologists. The imbalanced ratio in Engelhardt's trip, for Fox and Swazey, is between agency and purpose. While Engelhardt shares with Fox and Swazey the *purpose* of understanding how the viewpoint of the Chinese responds to moral dilemmas in medicine, his method—or *agency*—is misaligned. As Fox and Swazey put it, his "cultural myopia" prevents him from being able to see how morality organizes Chinese medicine, even when it is plainly in view.

Fox and Swazey's depiction of Engelhardt's "myopia" is akin to what Burke refers to as "trained incapacity," the inability to see aspects of the world because we have been trained (in Engelhardt's case philosophically) in a manner that disables our ability to see alternative perspectives. In the next part of their essay, Fox and Swazey describe the "Chinese medical morality" they were able to discover using their ethnographic skills—and which Engelhardt, lacking that capacity, had missed.

But it would be a mistake to view Fox and Swazey's essay as primarily about China. By beginning with their account and criticism of Engelhardt, they indicate what the real subject of this essay is: the trained incapacity of American bioethicists in general. Fox and Swazey are arguing that Engelhardt misunderstood China, but the account of that misunderstanding encapsulates the general inability of bioethics to be a true expression of medical morality in the context of American society. As they charge:

> In our sociological view, the paradigm of values and beliefs, and of reflections on them, that has developed and been institutionalized in American bioethics is an impoverished and skewed expression of our society's cultural tradition. In a highly intellectualized but essentially fundamentalistic way, it thins out the fullness of that tradition and bends it away from some of the deepest sources of its meaning and vitality.[40]

The fundamental trouble in bioethics for Fox and Swazey is that it lacks the appropriate agency—that is, sociological methods—for responding to the scene of American society. Without this intellectual equipment, bioethics will continue to respond to moral problems with a profound poverty of understanding morality in medicine. For Fox and Swazey, the anecdote of Engelhardt's travels (especially in comparison to their own sociological journey) expresses the essential problem with bioethics in America.

JAMES DRANE AND THE LACK OF IMBALANCE

James Drane begins his essay "Character and the Moral Life: A Virtue Approach to Biomedical Ethics" by quoting a story from James Gustafson's *Can Ethics Be Christian?*. In that book, Gustafson recounts the time he was in a bar with an academic colleague and they witness a "rather drunken soldier" being cheated by the bartender, resulting in an altercation. Noting that the soldier is too drunk to return home, Gustafson and his friend are able to ascertain his address from his wallet; they use some of the soldier's money to arrange for a cab to take him home. They write a note stating what they had done and who they were, including information about how to contact them if the soldier or his family wished to get more details. They also inform the cab driver that they have the soldier's address and know how much money was left in his wallet, so they will be able to confirm that the soldier and his possessions arrive home safely.

It seems strange to begin an essay on virtue in bioethics with a case that has nothing to do with medicine, much less with bioethics. Drane acknowledges as much but asserts that the actions taken in the story "could serve as a model for the character and virtues of a good physician."[41] If this story is a representative anecdote, as I believe it is, it is an unusual one, for one could argue that there really is no imbalance in terms of Bruner's model. Offering assistance to a stranger drunk in a bar seems to be an act in harmony with the scene, agency, purpose, attitude, and agent. I contend, however, that the lack of an imbalance in the narrative is the exception that proves the rule, for Drane's essay is fundamentally a critique of bioethics for not focusing on character. In the Gustafson story, the term that has dominance over the other terms is that of the agent. And this is why the narrative acts as a representative anecdote against traditional theory in bioethics: if the agent is of good character, Drane is arguing, there will be no imbalance. Good character ensures that the correct action will be taken in the correct place with the correct purpose, attitude, and agency.

Drane's representative anecdote is better understood through Burke's original pentadic analysis than through Bruner's, for what is important in the narrative is not the cause of Trouble but the reason for balance. In Burke's model, our descriptions betray what we believe are the motives for human actions, and Drane seeks to bring attention back to the humans doing those actions. The problem with traditional bioethics, according to Drane, is that it "is focused mainly on quandaries and dilemmas generated by discrete acts," and so the discipline spends its energy and time on "finding appropriate abstract principles and rules to apply to particular quandaries."[42] The Gustafson narrative represents an ethic that is neither quandary-based nor dependent on context. As a representative anecdote, it suggests that the point is not how to solve a series of specific problems but how to respond with the appropriate action in all situations, based on character.

Drane's emphasis on agency is a corrective to bioethics' misguided emphasis on various imbalances in medicine. As Drane himself acknowledges, the Gustafson narrative "illustrates better than any argument that character and virtue in many situations are more important than methodologies of moral reasoning, rules, principles, rights, and the like."[43] Its lack of imbalance is its argument.

CONCLUSION

While in our examination of retrodiction we attended to the grand narratives of bioethics and how they are constructed to serve a general argument, this chapter has focused on the use of the anecdotal, which can have as much rhetorical power to direct an issue as historical framing. As mentioned above, the importance of the representative anecdote is the manner in which it "synecdochically represents" a larger text.[44] In Bruner's extension of Burke's model, we can see that this synecdochical representation also entails a reproduction of the moral imbalance that the bioethicist sees in the biomedical world. Constructing a narrative that has a particular pentadic imbalance becomes a compelling way to subtly direct the reader to anticipate, as does historical plotting, a particular corrective to that imbalance. After all, bioethics is not interested in simply indicating the presence of moral problems, but also in providing directions for the rewriting of those narratives. In the next chapter on dissociation, we turn away from the rhetorical use of narrative toward a different type of redescription, as a way to describe moral problems in a manner that creates new divisions. We will investigate how, in their attempts to make an argument, bioethicists recategorize the world.

NOTES

1. Barry Brummett, "Burke's Representative Anecdote as a Method in Media Criticism," *Critical Studies in Mass Communication* 1, no. 2 (2009): 163.
2. Arnie Madsen, "Burke's Representative Anecdote as a Critical Method," in *Extensions of the Burkean System*, ed. James W. Cheseboro (Tuscaloosa, AL: University of Alabama Press, 1993), 210–211.
3. Kenneth Burke, *A Grammar of Motives* (Berkeley, CA: University of California Press, 1969), xv.
4. See Floyd D. Anderson, "Five Fingers or Six? Pentad or Hexad?," *KB Journal* 6, no. 2 (2010), https://kbjournal.org/anderson.

5. As quoted in Kenneth Burke, "Questions and Answers About the Pentad," *College Composition and Communication* 29, no. 4 (1978): 332.

6. Burke, "Questions and Answers About the Pentad," 332.

7. Burke, "Questions and Answers About the Pentad," 332.

8. Alexis M. May and E. David Klonsky, "What Distinguishes Suicide Attempters from Suicide Ideators? A Meta-Analysis of Potential Factors," *Clinical Psychology: Science and Practice* 23, no. 1 (2016): 5–20.

9. Glenn Graber, "The Rationality of Suicide," in *Suicide and Euthanasia: The Rights of Personhood*, ed. Albin Eser and Samuel E. Wallace (Knoxville, TN: University of Tennessee Press, 1981).

10. Margaret Pabst Battin, *The Death Debate: Ethical Issues in Suicide* (Upper Saddle River, NJ: Prentice Hall, 1996).

11. Emile Durkheim, *On Suicide*, trans. Robin Buss (London: Penguin, 2006).

12. David A. Ling, "A Pentadic Analysis of Senator Edward Kennedy's Address to the People of Massachusetts, July 25, 1969," *Communication Studies* 21, no. 2 (1970): 80–86.

13. Barry Brummett, "A Pentadic Analysis of Ideologies in Two Gay Rights Controversies," *Central States Speech Journal* 30, no. 3 (1979): 250–261.

14. Cyd C. Ropp, "Pentadic Cartography: Mapping Obstetric Medicine and Traditional Midwifery" (Paper presented at the National Communication Association, New Orleans, LA, November 2002).

15. Tod Chambers, "Framing Our Mistakes," in *Margin of Error: The Necessity, Inevitability, and Ethics of Mistakes in Medicine and Bioethics Consultation*, ed. Susan Rubin and Laurie Zoloth (Frederick, MD: University Publishing Group, 2000), 13–24.

16. David Blakesley, *The Elements of Dramatism* (New York: Longman, 2002) 32.

17. Jerome S. Bruner, *Actual Minds, Possible Worlds* (Cambridge, MA: Harvard University Press, 1986), 20.

18. Jerome Bruner, "The Narrative Construction of Reality," *Critical Inquiry* 18, no. 1 (Autumn 1991): 16.

19. Anthony G. Amsterdam and Jerome S. Bruner, *Minding the Law* (Cambridge, MA: Harvard University Press, 2000) 130.

20. See H. Porter Abbott, *The Cambridge Introduction to Narrative* (Cambridge; New York: Cambridge University Press, 2002), 12–14.

21. Matthew T. Althouse and Floyd D. Anderson, "'Trouble with a Capital T': Jerome S. Bruner's Reenvisioning of Kenneth Burke's Dramatistic Pentad," *K.B. Journal* 11, no. 2 (Spring 2016). http://www.kbjournal.org/althouse-anderson, 1.

22. Bruner, *Actual Minds, Possible Worlds*, 19–21.

23. Althouse and Anderson, "'Trouble with a Capital T': Jerome S. Bruner's Reenvisioning of Kenneth Burke's Dramatistic Pentad," 6.

24. John Cash, "The Case Study as Representative Anecdote," in *Case Studies and the Dissemination of Knowledge*, ed. Joy Damousi, Birgit Lang, and Katie Sutton (New York: Routledge, 2015), 31–48.

25. Albert R. Jonsen, Mark Siegler, and William J. Winslade, *Clinical Ethics: A Practical Approach to Ethical Decisions in Clinical Medicine*, 3rd ed. (New York: McGraw-Hill Health Professions Division, 1992), 4–10.

26. Jonsen, Siegler, and Winslade, *Clinical Ethics: A Practical Approach to Ethical Decisions in Clinical Medicine*, 8.

27. Ezekiel J. Emanuel, *The Ends of Human Life: Medical Ethics in a Liberal Polity* (Cambridge, MA: Harvard University Press, 1991) 6.

28. Emanuel, *The Ends of Human Life: Medical Ethics in a Liberal Polity*, 3.

29. Emanuel, *The Ends of Human Life: Medical Ethics in a Liberal Polity*, 5.

30. Emanuel, *The Ends of Human Life: Medical Ethics in a Liberal Polity*, 4.

31. Emanuel, *The Ends of Human Life: Medical Ethics in a Liberal Polity*, 245.

32. Jodi Halpern, *From Detached Concern to Empathy: Humanizing Medical Practice* (Oxford: Oxford University Press, 2001), 4.

33. Halpern, *From Detached Concern to Empathy: Humanizing Medical Practice*, 4.

34. Halpern, *From Detached Concern to Empathy: Humanizing Medical Practice*, 144.

35. Hilde Lindemann Nelson, *Damaged Identities, Narrative Repair* (Ithaca, NY: Cornell University Press, 2001), 3.

36. Lindemann Nelson, *Damaged Identities, Narrative Repair*, 5.

37. Lindemann Nelson, *Damaged Identities, Narrative Repair*, 5.

38. Lindemann Nelson, *Damaged Identities, Narrative Repair*, 175.

39. Renée C. Fox and Judith P. Swazey, "Medical Morality Is Not Bioethics: Medical Ethics in China and the United States," *Perspectives in Biology and Medicine* 27 (1984): 337.

40. Fox and Swazey, "Medical Morality Is Not Bioethics: Medical Ethics in China and the United States," 358.

41. James F. Drane, "Character and the Moral Life: A Virtue Approach to Biomedical Ethics," in *A Matter of Principles?: Ferment in U.S. Bioethics*, ed. E. R. DuBose, R. P. Hamel, and L. J. O'Connel (Valley Forge, PA: Trinity, 1994), 184.

42. Drane, "Character and the Moral Life: A Virtue Approach to Biomedical Ethics," 285.

43. Drane, "Character and the Moral Life: A Virtue Approach to Biomedical Ethics," 287.

44. Madsen, "Burke's Representative Anecdote as a Critical Method," 210.

Chapter 4

Dissociation

In the chapter on retrodiction, I discussed the historical frame created by Stephen Toulmin and Albert Jonsen. I mentioned that in the prologue to *The Abuse of Casuistry*, the authors reference a shared personal experience, their observation of the work of the National Commission for the Protection of Human Subjects of Biomedical and Behavioral Research. Their fundamental insight from this experience was that the commission was successful in thinking through the moral problems they were charged with resolving only as long as they attended to particular cases. In other words, the group's agreement on how to resolve the various cases was possible not when they appealed to broader moral principles, but when they disregarded them. Jonsen and Toulmin have cited this experience in a number of other publications as well. Toulmin recounts it in the essays "The Tyranny of Principles"[1] and "How Medicine Saved the Life of Ethics";[2] Jonsen includes it in "Casuistry and Clinical Ethics"[3] and "Casuistry: An Alternative or Complement to Principles?"[4] For both of these bioethicists, the experience is a key representative anecdote. The imbalance in the story is between purpose and agency. Jonsen and Toulmin argue that what the representatives on the commission thought their purpose was—to apply general principles to individual moral problems—was incongruent with how they actually accomplished the task: the creation of a theory-free (or, according to John Arras' critique, a theory-light[5]) taxonomy. For these two proponents of a revival of casuistry, this imbalance encapsulates the central problem with contemporary bioethics. That is, we think we need principles to resolve moral problems, but more often than not they end up blocking a resolution rather than facilitating one. The representative anecdote also contains Jonsen and Toulmin's solution to the problem—to decouple principles from the method of bioethics.

In making this argument, Jonsen and Toulmin use a rhetorical move that Chaim Perelman and Lucie Olbrechts-Tyteca refer to as *dissociation.* Dissociation is a rhetorical scheme in which elements that were thought to be a single entity are redescribed as fundamentally distinct. Perelman and Olbrechts-Tyteca believe that, in philosophical thought, "original" work tends to come from dissociation. Their prototypical example, one of the first and most durable instances of dissociation in Western philosophy, is the disjoining of appearance from reality. In fact, they argue, this division is so central to philosophy that "[r]easoning by dissociation is characterized from the start by the opposition of appearance and reality";[6] this pairing can be found "directly or indirectly in all dissociations" in philosophical discourse.[7] Frans van Eemeren et al. write that this particular conceptual split results in one of the parts becoming "associated with the *apparent* (i.e., the peripheral or false aspect of the original single concept) and the other with the *real* (i.e., the central or true aspect of the original single concept)."[8] In doing so, this split does not result in two equal parts but instead in a hierarchical binary in which the "real" is valued over the "apparent." The classic illustration is when Plato dissociates the physical appearance of the world from its Forms, which hold the greater reality. Such a hierarchy can also be reversed, as Alan Gross and Ray Dearin observe. They contrast Platonic idealism with the philosophy of Maurice Merleau-Ponty, which asserts that the apparent, or phenomenological, is more real than the ideal.[9]

In both examples, the dissociation consists of two key moves. First, writes Kathryn Olson, is the "differentiating and hierarchically arranging [of] usually two elements of a single concept"; next, "the rhetoric portrays one element as positive and more highly valued, simultaneously devaluing another element by assigning to it the negative qualities of the formerly unified concept."[10] Using this insight, we see that when Jonsen and Toulmin argue for the dissociation of principles from moral reasoning, they are essentially arguing for the superiority of casuistry over principle-based approaches. Indeed, in "The Tyranny of Principles" Toulmin concludes his commentary on the National Commission anecdote by stating that principles really had nothing to do with the process of moral decision-making; their true role was "to square the collective ethical conclusions of the Commission as a whole with each individual commissioner's other *non*ethical commitments."[11]

Yet in ethics, as we see in Merleau-Ponty's reversal of the typical privileging of reality over appearance, any dissociation can itself become a part of another dissociation—and Toulmin's de-linking of principles from bioethics is no exception. Edmund Pincoffs begins his essay "Quandary Ethics" with a series of quotes, the first of which is from Toulmin: "Ethics is everybody's concern . . . Everyone . . . is faced with moral problems—problems about which, after more or less reflection, a decision must be reached." This quote comes from the beginning of what is perhaps one of Toulmin's most influential works, *Reason in Ethics*.[12] Like his work in casuistry with Jonsen, one finds that Toulmin saw the resolution of moral problems as the key subject of ethical analysis. It is for this reason that Toulmin makes the claim that "medicine saved the life of ethics" by forcing philosophers to move away from a focus on rules and instead attend to cases.[13] Interestingly, one finds in this essay arguing for the power of medicine to save this neglected specialty in philosophy that Toulmin retells the story of the National Commission for the Protection of Human Subjects and Behavioral Research. Pincoffs, quoting Toulmin (as well as Hare, Brandt, and Singer), illustrates how ethics has come to be understood as focused on the resolution of moral problems. In his essay, Pincoffs argues that this focus is profoundly misguided. Reaching back to ancient Greek philosophy, he makes a historical appeal for the dissociation of ethics and problem-solving, noting that ethical explorations centered on the matter of (permanent, perfectible) character, not (ephemeral, mundane) problem-solving. Pincoffs is careful to acknowledge that resolving moral problems is a part of ethics—just a very narrow part. The larger questions concern character, something deeper and greater than any particular choice made in response to any particular quandary. And in this differentiation, Pincoffs creates a hierarchy in which the understanding of ethics proposed by Jonsen and Toulmin is made into the lower form—something secondary to the *real* question of character. After all, a case asks us to come to a decision irrespective of the particular person being confronted with the problem. Yet for Pincoffs, answering the question of how one should act requires that we first ask who the particular person is who will be acting. In the end, he pronounces, "it does not follow that because my decision would have been right for anyone in the same circumstances it would have been right for me."[14]

The debates described above feature bioethicists using dissociation to advocate for one of the existing methods of practice (casuistry, principlism, virtue ethics). But dissociation has also been used to generate entirely new theoretical approaches. Care ethics, for example, is based on the belief that there is a fundamental split between two "voices," the voice of care and the voice of justice. Seeing these two perspectives in simultaneous tension, rather than one (the voice of care) as an early and immature version of the later, wiser one (justice), was a revision of Lawrence Kohlberg's original formulation of moral development. In Kohlberg's schema, the key features of the care perspective were designated as early stages of a more mature perspective, and this early stage largely described the moral reasoning of women, which tended to stay focused on interpersonal relationships. As Carol Gilligan explains in *In a Different Voice*, "Prominent among those who thus appear to be deficient in moral development when measured by Kohlberg's scale are women, whose judgments seem to exemplify the third stage of his six-stage sequence."[15] Gilligan's revisioning of Kohlberg's conclusion was not that the features of the care perspective were a stage in development, but a separate and equally mature form of moral deliberation. (Gilligan's early work on the care orientation even included her own series of stages of moral development. While she later moved away from this formulation, I mention it here to emphasize how the care perspective was originally viewed by Gilligan as a distinct whole, fully as complete as Kohlberg's.) As with other instances of dissociation, the two gendered spheres are seen by care ethics proponents as separate—but not equal. Due to the nature and purpose of health care, and health-care ethics in particular,[16] the care orientation is considered superior to the justice orientation. As Alisa Carse observes in an essay on the importance of care ethics in the education of health-care professionals, an emphasis on the justice orientation "may run the risk of encouraging a coarseness of feeling a lack of care and compassion necessary to fostering hope and ensuring that a patient's good is served in the healing process."[17]

DISSOCIATION BY DEFINITION

A good deal of the history of the discipline of bioethics has been dedicated to acts of definition, for example, life, futility, personhood, capacity. As Perelman and Olbrechts-Tyteca observe, definition serves as "an instrument of the dissociation of concepts" used to bolster novel philosophical claims by providing "the real, true meaning of the concept as opposed to its customary or apparent usage."[18] Definitions enable the bioethicist to argue for the priority of a new approach, theory, or method by dissociating characteristics which were viewed as essential in a prior argument. Perelman and Olbrechts-Tyteca note that a "statement that something falls or does not fall within a given concept amounts to the indirect introduction of a dissociative definition, especially when the introduction of a new characteristic becomes the criterion for the correct use of the concept."[19] To control a definition is, in turn to control the argument.

In "Arguing About Definitions," Edward Schiappa shows that when an argument invokes the "real definition" of something, dissociation is almost always the rhetorical foundation. Yet Schiappa calls arguments that rely upon dissociation-by-definition "dysfunctional." The example that Schiappa analyzes is the modern redefinition of death as based solely on brain activity. In his look at the various attempts to provide a "real definition" of death, as opposed to a pragmatic one, Schiappa concludes that such arguments are "dysfunctional to the extent that they direct attention to 'is' claims and away from 'ought' claims."[20] Schiappa notes that the debate over death was the result of technological advances in medicine that permitted heart and lung activity after the loss of all brain function. In the examples that Schiappa analyzes, it is clear that there is an active attempt to dissociate death from the activity (or lack of activity) of the heart and lungs. In these arguments, the brain becomes defined as the true locus of personhood, and so the loss of personhood, in turn, represents death—even if the body is otherwise capable of being biologically maintained. One illustration is Henry Beecher's assertion, following the report of the Harvard ad hoc committee on the concept of brain death,[21] that the

> definition of irreversible coma we set down has been widely accepted . . . as a workable definition of *death*, not death of the heart, so dear to some lawyers . . . but, of much more consequence, as a definition of the irreversible termination of the personality, the death of the brain, death indeed.[22]

In this statement Beecher dissociates the definition of death from the death of the heart—and even from a purely biological state. It is not simply that the brain's function is more relevant than the heart's, but that the brain is the very locus of the person.

As Schiappa glosses Perelman and Olbrechts-Tyteca, "a dissociative definition is at work when a characteristic becomes the criterion of the correct use of the concept."[23] The effect of establishing this new criterion is to exclude alternative and thus competing definitions. For example, in "On the Definition and Criterion of Death," James Bernat, Charles Culver, and Bernard Gert replace Beecher's putatively subjective criterion of *personhood* (as seen in Beecher's argument) with the physical, "objective" criterion of whole brain function. As they see it, the loss of the functioning of the whole brain "is perfectly correlated with the permanent cessation of function of the organism as a whole because the brain is necessary for the functioning of the organism as a whole."[24] Bernat, Culver, and Gert dissociate death from a locus in the heart and lungs, but also from any conceptualization they argue is "not biological." Any definition that entails "certain kinds of abilities and qualities of awareness" is insufficient, subjective, and "inherently vague."[25] In this argument Bernat, Culver, and Gert wish to dissociate a definition of death from the subjective definitions related to personhood as well as from objective definitions that relate it to any other part of the human body.

Dissociation, Henry Johnstone notes, does not follow any general logical pattern; "there is only the logic of each particular dissociation, generated in each case by a particular problem."[26] Yet whether by anecdote, schema, or definition, dissociation permits the bioethicist to redescribe an issue or debate and thereby effect, as Perelman and Olbrechts-Tyteca characterize it, a "profound change in the conceptual data that are used as the basis of argument."[27] Perelman and Olbrechts-Tyteca also identify a rhetorical move that does *not* change the data so profoundly and which should be distinguished from dissociation. They call this more modest approach the "breaking of connecting links."[28]

BREAKING CONNECTING LINKS IN BIOETHICS

According to Perelman and Olbrechts-Tyteca, dissociation "assumes the original unity of elements comprised within a single conception and designated by a single notion."[29] Breaking the links differs in that no prior unity obtains; it means arguing "that elements which should remain separate and independent have been improperly associated."[30] A good illustration from within bioethics discourse can be found in Tom Beauchamp and James Childress' separation of beneficence and nonmaleficence, which they believe were misconstrued as a single entity in the *Belmont Report.*

Issued in 1978, the *Belmont Report* famously promoted three "basic ethical principles" that were used to justify positions for research ethics: respect for persons, beneficence, and justice. At the same time the *Belmont Report* was being written, Beauchamp and Childress were at work on their foundational book, *The Principles of Biomedical Ethics*, first published in 1979. According to Beauchamp, it was a common mistake to think that the *Belmont Report*'s framework was the "starting point"[31] for the *Principles.* One significant difference between the two was the number of proposed principles—the *Report* identified three, as cited above, while Beauchamp and Childress named four. Beauchamp and Childress' principles were apparently similar to those of the *Report*—they included beneficence, nonmaleficence, respect for autonomy, and justice—but, as Beauchamp explains,

> I thought at the time, and still do, that the National Commission was confused in the way it delineated the principle of respect for persons. It seemed to blend two independent principles: a principle of respect for autonomy and a principle of protecting and avoiding the causation of harm to incompetent persons.

He and his co-author "both thought that we should stick to our thesis that the principle of beneficence must be distinguished from the principle of nonmaleficence, though the National Commission failed to make any such distinction."[32] In this example, Beauchamp and Childress are not proposing a radical split within the traditional notion of beneficence or of nonmaleficence, nor are they arguing that either is something essentially different than a principle (both of which would be acts of dissociation). Instead, they are saying that separate principles have been merged incorrectly. This false link must be broken.

Another example of breaking connecting links can be found in the debate over the American Academy of Pediatrics' (AAP) recommendations that a child's opinion on a health-care matter be given greater importance as the child matures. The AAP separates children into three distinct categories: those who do not have decision-making capacity, those developing capacity, and those who have capacity. In *The Hastings Report*, Lainie Ross questions a number of aspects of the AAP argument, but her major concern is in relation to cases where parents and children disagree. While she concedes the AAP's position that some children have decision-making capacity, she argues that capacity is simply one small part of what would be necessary to grant children decision-making power. In particular, she asserts, no child has had adequate time "in which to develop 'enabling virtues'—habits, including the habit of self-control, which advance their lifetime autonomy and opportunities."[33] In taking the AAP to task for improperly associating the abilities of adults with that of children via the concept of "competency," Ross breaks this link and reaffirms the difference between the abilities of children and those of adults.

It is often noted that the development of bioethics in the United States hinged on bringing those normally thought to be outside of medicine—philosophers, theologians, sociologists, lawyers—into the clinical environment to help resolve problems.[34] In "Clinical Ethics and Clinical Medicine," an editorial published in the *Archives of Internal Medicine*, Mark Siegler attacks this very mix. "Interdisciplinary efforts are laudable" in general, he allows, but constructing a field focused on medicine but dominated by nonphysicians is wrong.[35] The experts to whom the practice is being applied "have had only limited involvement in its development,"[36] while the nonphysicians and nonscientists leading the field "represent interests that are quite different from those of the medical-scientific community."[37]

Siegler's editorial both takes aim at the improper blending of insider and outsider and brightens the line dividing the two. Coining an acronym for the interdisciplinary field—BME (biomedical ethics)—he discusses its rise via the creation of new journals, departments, and graduate programs. Noting that some in BME have "actually expressed their disdain for traditional, Hippocratic, bedside medical ethics,"[38] and citing Robert Veatch as one of the sources for this disdain, he lays out his argument for a new ethical field, one that is an organic part of medical practice: "clinical ethics." It is at this point that he leans into the distinction between BME and clinical ethics. Practitioners of BME are mere observers; they "rely on the counterfeit courage of the noncombatant."[39] Further, they can never truly understand the consequences of the decisions they advise. In what could be thought of as a representative anecdote, Siegler quotes a parable by Søren Kierkegaard in which the Danish philosopher asks us to imagine a pilot of a ship who has never actually been to sea. When the pilot encounters a storm for the first time, he knows what to do technically, but he is unprepared for the terror and fear of applying that technical knowledge in the real world: he is a stranger to what Kierkegaard calls "the change that takes place in the knower when he has to apply his knowledge."[40] With this story, Siegler wishes to break the connecting links that were constructed between ethicists outside the medical profession (the callow pilots) and those within it (the meaningfully experienced). Insisting on the eternal outsider status of the nonphysician—who could only achieve Kierkegaard's deeper knowledge if they too practiced medicine—Siegler returns medical ethics to the realm of self-regulation. BME proponents have incorrectly associated the authority of the nonphysician with that of the physician, the only figure who has a true understanding of medicine and its moral foundations, and thus medicine's only legitimate source of oversight or guidance. In this, Siegler is arguing that the modern bioethics movement has as one of its prime convictions that the moral philosopher is as warranted to make moral assessments as the physician who must live with the consequences of a decision. Siegler wishes to break this connecting link that has been created so that the morality of medicine should only be determined by those who are engaged in the practice of medicine and not the "noncombatants" of BME.

In my discussion of anagnorisis, I began the chapter by looking at the way Peter Singer argues against speciesism. Singer believes that the distinctions we should be concerned with are not between humans and other animals, but between different types of consciousness and interests. This orientation eliminates what he sees as a false distinction between humans and animals. A more vital distinction for Singer than the one between humans and animals is the one between humans and apes versus mollusks and insects. In "Rights, Animal and Human," David Carlin refuses the arguments of those, like Singer, who wish to dissolve the difference between the human animal and all other species. He acknowledges that "there *is* only a narrow gap between humans the highest of the animals"[41]—yet it is still a meaningful one, one that must be maintained. To dissolve this distinction is "anti-Christian," Carlin contends, for it would overturn the fundamental notion that humans are created in the image of God and thus "reduce human nature to nothing more than its biological status."[42] Overall, Carlin's argument against granting animals the same rights as humans is meant to preserve a distinction he believes has been wrongly eroded in an otherwise valid attempt to argue for the humane treatment of animals.

DISSOCIATING ABORTION FROM THE DEFINITION OF PERSONHOOD

One of the most famous thought experiments in moral philosophy was created by Judith Jarvis Thomson in her "A Defense of Abortion."

Thomson begins her essay by addressing one of the most common arguments against abortion: that a fetus has the same status as a human person. While she believes that the claim that a fetus has this status at the moment of conception is not persuasive, she acknowledges that at some point during pregnancy, the fetus is likely to be considered to have this status. But then her argument takes a remarkable turn. She goes ahead and grants the argument that, at conception, a fetus is a person, with all of the rights attendant on such a designation. The reader might assume that, after this acknowledgment, the debate over abortion has been concluded, and Thomson will now agree that, in all cases, abortion must be considered immoral. Instead, it is here that Thomson proposes her thought experiment.

Thomson asks us to imagine that we wake up one morning to find that we have been kidnapped by the Society of Music Lovers: we are a donor match for a very sick, very famous violinist, and the Society has surgically secured us to this violinist. Our kidneys are being used to provide this musician with the necessary medical treatment he will require for nine months, after which he will be healthy enough to live without the constant use of our organs.

> The director of the hospital now tells you, "Look, we're sorry the Society of Music Lovers did this to you—we would never have permitted it if we had known. But still, they did it, and the violinist now is plugged into you. To unplug you would be to kill him. But never mind, it's only for nine months. By then he will have recovered from his ailment, and can safely be unplugged from you." Is it morally incumbent on you to accede to this situation? No doubt it would be very nice of you if you did, a great kindness. But do you *have* to accede to it? What if it were not nine months, but nine years? Or longer still? What if the director of the hospital says, "Tough luck, I agree, but you've now got to stay in bed, with the violinist plugged into you, for the rest of your life. Because remember this. All persons have a right to life, and violinists are persons. Granted you have a right to decide what happens in and to your body, but a person's right to life outweighs your right to decide what happens in and to your body. So you cannot ever be unplugged from him." I imagine you would regard this as outrageous, which suggests that something really is wrong with that plausible-sounding argument I mentioned a moment ago.[43]

In this hypothetical, Thomson dissociates the issue of abortion from the moral status of the fetus. Setting aside the "conceptual data" that was thought to be the heart of the argument, Thomson is able to effect a "profound change" in the debate—while it may be admirable to sustain another person's life with our own bodies, society would never impose this as an absolute obligation on everyone. In her argument, both the violinist and the fetus have full status as humans; still, she claims, no individual person is obliged to serve as another person's agent of life, even for a limited period of time.

In the abortion debate, the notion of the decision to terminate a pregnancy and the question of the moral status of the fetus are seen as a single whole. Thomson is able, through this thought experiment, to dissociate the two. This dissociation creates a new hierarchy in which the principle of personal liberty takes priority over the definition of personhood. Pregnancy becomes a voluntary activity in this transformation of the debate into an issue of social contract. In turn, the question of continuing a pregnancy becomes, in a liberal society, a supererogatory act rather than a required obligation.

DISSOCIATING ENHANCEMENT TECHNOLOGY FROM MEDICAL PROFESSIONALISM

An ongoing debate in medicine is whether we can distinguish treatment from enhancement. From reconstructive surgery to growth hormones to psychiatric medications that make one "better than well," there has been a general critique of interventions that may exceed the duty of medical professionals to return people to health. This critique holds that medicine is never meant to make a patient superior to the average person.

Erik Parens addresses the treatment/enhancement distinction within bioethics in his essay "Is Better Always Good?," which summarizes the conclusions of a project at the Hastings Center on enhancement technology.[44] He notes that in the enhancement debate, one finds two different conversations, which at times overlap, concerning the ethics of enhancement technology. One of the conversations explores whether such technology "would be undermining extra-medical, social goals or would be exacerbating already existing social problems";[45] the other considers whether this technology should be permitted within the medical system.

This second conversation takes into account the general moral duties of health-care professionals and the matter of funding; should society fund enhancement measures under the umbrella of healthcare? After recounting some of the positions that have been adopted in this second conversation, Parens introduces a concept that he credits to the philosopher Jamie Nelson: "schmocters." Nelson herself derives this concept from the practice in philosophical circles of adding "schm" to a word when it resembles another entity but is distinct in some specific way. This idea is often credited to Saul Kripke's notion of "schmidentity," which he discusses in his book *Naming and Necessity*.[46] Parens asks readers to imagine there is a community of practitioners called schmocters, who practice what they refer to as schmedicine. They may resemble doctors in terms of their technical skill, but their customs are different. They are "expert in using new biotechnologies to enhance human capacities and traits, and they sell their expertise to willing, indeed, enthusiastic purchasers."[47] These alternative technicians of the human body do not rely on any form of insurance, and instead work purely fee-for-service.

The introduction of this hypothetical profession dissociates the enhancement debate from the traditional goals of medicine and, in doing so, eliminates the need to make a distinction between enhancement and medicine. As Parens observes, the very goals of being a schmoctor set aside the moral goals of medicine because the only goals that concern schmocters are the goals of schmedicine. It could be argued that, with this dissociation, Parens shifts the enhancement debate from the realm of medical professional responsibility to that of political science. That is, with the practice of schmedicine being a thriving business, the new debate would be over the degree to which society limits a person's choice to transform their body. Thus, while Parens seems to resolve this part of the enhancement debate in terms of the goals of medicine, the issues concerning what he refers to as the "goals of society" are even more complex than before.

As medicine changes in terms of its training and goals, it sometimes seeks to separate itself from issues that have traditionally been considered under its ethical purview. As in Parens' enhancement/medicine dissociation, the extraction of an issue from the discussion about professional duty can be used to address a number of long-standing quandaries in medicine. In their essay "License to Kill: A New Model for Excusing Medically Assisted Dying?," Richard Huxtable and Jonathan Ives argue for the permissibility of assistance in dying by physicians by advocating for a new subspeciality they refer to as thanatologists.[48] Their argument is, in some measure a response to an essay by Willard Gaylin, Leon Kass, Edmund Pellegrino, and Mark Siegler titled "Doctors Must Not Kill,"[49] in which the authors claim that if physicians were to be involved in causing the death of their patients, it would result in a "collapse" of medicine's "moral center," for those physicians would "never again be worthy of trust and respect as healer[s] and protector[s] of life in all its frailty."[50] Huxtable and Ives counter that this apocalyptic possibility can be averted by limiting medically assisted dying to a single (highly regulated) specialty within medicine. Their argument does not rely on the kind of dissociation we saw in Parens, who sought to redescribe enhancement as an occupation entirely outside of medicine. In opting not to separate thanatology from medicine, their argument skirts the concerns of Gaylin et al. instead of fully answering them. Huxtable and Ives claim that, by creating this new subspecialty, "a clear message will be sent to the public, and to the profession, that there will remain a clear distinction between those professionals who will be involved in assisting death, and those who will not and cannot"[51]—yet a more potent argument could be made by dissociating the medical profession's involvement entirely from this action. After all, doing so would circumvent any attack on assisted dying that is based on the traditionally understood goals of the medical profession.

In some ways, the dissociation of medicine from questions long considered matters of medical ethics is captured by John Lantos in his book *Do We Still Need Doctors?* For Lantos, changes in medicine necessitate changes in moral responsibility. If we dissociate the medical profession from a moral problem, he observes, the problem does not somehow go away; it simply becomes a political problem. As Lantos notes, the presence in bioethics of nonphysicians has also brought with it questions of dissociation related to medical practice and the medical profession. That is, if we think of physicians as solely technicians of the body, their expertise "as morally neutral as that of electricians or auto mechanics,"[52] then what they are permitted to do to those bodies is not for them to decide, but a question for the larger society. And in a purely libertarian political world, that question would already be answered: with the individual's permission, anything could be done to anyone.

DISSOCIATING DEAFNESS FROM DISABILITY

Robert Sparrow begins his essay on the ethics of cochlear implants by stating, "'Cochlear implants' are a technology which attempts to 'cure' deafness by bypassing the outer ear through electrical stimulation of the auditory nerve."[53] In that sentence, quotation marks are placed around two parts—"cochlear implants" and "cure"—but the two sets are used for very different reasons. The first set of quotation marks is used to indicate the introduction of a technical term. The second set, around the word "cure," is meant not to introduce a neutral technology but to debunk the perception of its nature. The term "cure" requires the notion of a disease or affliction—a prerequisite with which Sparrow strongly disagrees. In some ways, Sparrow's entire argument is captured in this single opening sentence. As Sparrow goes on to argue, hearing persons could not imagine that anyone, especially a Deaf person, would not experience the loss of hearing as a "tragic loss and a disability" and, Sparrow imagines, a hearing person who considers anyone who does not hold this view as "perverse."[54] The dissociation of Deafness from the category of disability has in fact been a powerful form of critique against the use of cochlear implants.[55]

One of the initial criticisms of cochlear implants was that the technology did not provide an adequate simulation of the experience of hearing by a non-deaf person. This form of argument against cochlear implants was understandably weakened as the technology of the implants improved. The stronger argument against the implants resides in rejecting them even if the implants achieve an experience of hearing equal to that of a non-Deaf person. This argument, which is made by Sparrow and others, relies on dissociation. Disability assumes that there has been some form of loss in ability; in the case of deafness, it is the loss of an ability that a healthy person possesses. Yet for Sparrow, this is a deficient understanding of the experience of Deafness. A better understanding is what Sparrow introduces as an "alternative model": Deafness not as the absence of an ability, but as an enhanced way of being. Deaf persons have superior abilities because of the way they communicate through sign language. Sparrow, for example, notes that Deaf people may "have a superior consciousness of subtlety of gesture and of the movement of bodies through space."[56] Sparrow also notes that in particular environments, such as those in which auditory noise can interfere with oral communication, Deaf people actually have an advantage. By dissociating Deafness from the notion of deficiency or loss and instead characterizing it as a different way of being in the world, Sparrow can denounce cochlear implants in the same manner one might denounce an attempt to change a person's ethnicity or race to fit the dominant culture. As Sparrow puts it,

> But if deafness is not a disability, what is it? At the heart of elements of the Deaf community's objection to cochlear implant technology is the claim that Deaf people constitute a minority culture rather than merely a group of people who share a disability.[57]

By dissociating deafness from disability, those who argue against cochlear implants are essentially arguing that the universal adoption of such technology is akin to an eradication of culture. The power of the argument resides in separating the experience of deafness as something to be treated as a medical condition and then, as in many instances of dissociation, presenting deafness in ways superior to other ways of being in the world.

DISSOCIATING SEX FROM PROCREATION

Gregory Pence, in *Who's Afraid of Human Cloning?,* argues for the moral permissibility of cloning humans. Throughout the book, Pence makes a number of arguments as to why cloning as a form of human reproduction should be considered acceptable. He attacks the "false seers of assisted human reproduction," noting that during the 1970s, a large number of bioethicists predicted catastrophic results from IVF. For Pence, the fact that these doom-filled predictions were incorrect should make us question similar statements about cloning, which he says have appeared in "waves" since IVF. He then attempts to dismantle the various misconceptions people have about what a human clone would be like in comparison to human beings created prior to this possibility.

In his sixth chapter, "Cloning and Sex," Pence takes on human cloning opponents who hold that sex and reproduction cannot be separated—and if they were to be, the social and moral consequences would be significant. He acknowledges the long tradition in Christianity of viewing reproduction as a necessary component of sexual relations. Two thinkers Pence addresses directly are Leon Kass and Gilbert Meilaender. Both see reproduction and sexuality as intertwined, and both see this whole as the basis of human civilization. Meilaender, a Protestant ethicist, ties his argument to interpretations of Biblical passages. Kass' proceeds from his belief that asexual reproduction is fundamentally contrary to the building blocks of human society. To permit reproduction without heterosexual relations would be to sacrifice the essential elements holding our society together.

Pence responds to this view with dissociation, simply refuting the moral entanglement presumed to bind sex with reproduction. He concludes his chapter by observing that cloning

> separates sex from reproduction, and, hence, symbolizes—in fact and concept—this break. As such, it resonates in our culture in a more emotional way than simply as a new way of making babies or as a new way of helping infertile couples. It appears that the separation of sex from reproduction strikes some deep fears in the human breast, making theological pundits predict that we are fast approaching reproductive Armageddon.[58]

For Pence, cloning as a form of asexual reproduction can be justified when we understand that the historical connection between the two is, in fact, a false unity. To dissociate sex from reproduction is to liberate both elements: "Sex is sex, and need not be anything more."[59] And so, sex becomes simply another way to reproduce, without any moral superiority over other forms of human creation, cloning included.

CONCLUSION

Dissociation is not simply a feature of the way bioethicists make arguments but a key feature of the discipline itself. Like the rhetorical methods discussed earlier, dissociation entails redescription; in depicting the world as comprising distinctions that were missed, it allows a moral debate to be radically reframed. Dissociation is never merely the observation of a hidden distinction but one that carries, in the act of redescription, an inherent value judgment. The classic philosophical dissociation of appearance and reality is in many ways the paradigm of this method, for within a perspective such as Platonism, these two entities do not hold equal value but instead form a hierarchy, with reality having greater importance than appearance. Similarly, in each of the dissociations discussed in this chapter, the described distinction allows the arguer to prioritize one of the two concepts. In Thomson's thought experiment, the debate on the origin of life comes second to the political liberty we should give to all people. In the enhancement debate, the issue is not as narrow as one of professionalism but a broader question about social justice. In the debate over cochlear implants, distinguishing Deafness from disability makes the question of a technological "fix" as problematic as the use of medicine to repair other social prejudices. By dissociating sex from reproduction, both acts can be freed from harmful constraints, such as a particular vision of family.

As Perelman and Olbrechts-Tyteca observe, all dissociation presupposes association. While this chapter has focused on the forms and effects of dissociation, in the next chapter, we will turn to the forms and effects of association—specifically those made through metaphor. Like dissociation, metaphor is a form of redescription in that it presents one concept through another.

NOTES

1. Stephen Toulmin, "The Tyranny of Principles," *Hastings Center Report* 11, no. 6 (1981): 31.
2. Stephen Toulmin, "How Medicine Saved the Life of Ethics," *Perspectives in Biology and Medicine* 25, no. 4 (Summer 1982): 741.
3. Albert R. Jonsen, "Casuistry and Clinical Ethics," *Theoretical Medicine* 7 (1986): 71.
4. Albert R. Jonsen, "Casuistry: An Alternative or Complement to Principles?," *Kennedy Institute of Ethics Journal* 5, no. 3 (1995): 239.
5. John D. Arras, "Getting Down to Cases: The Revival of Casuistry in Bioethics," *The Journal of Medicine and Philosophy* 16, no. 1 (February 1991): 29–51.
6. Chaïm Perelman, *The Realm of Rhetoric* (Notre Dame, IN: University of Notre Dame Press, 1982), 134.
7. Perelman, *The Realm of Rhetoric*, 126.
8. Frans H. van Eemeren et al., *Handbook of Argumentation Theory: A Critical Survey of Classical Backgrounds and Modern Studies* (Dordrecht: Springer, 1987), 282.
9. Alan G. Gross and Ray D. Dearin, *Chaim Perelman* (Albany, NY: State University of New York Press, 2003), 91.
10. Kathryn M. Olson, "Dissociation," in *Encyclopedia of Rhetoric and Composition: Communication from Ancient Times to the Information Age*, ed. Theresa Enos (New York: Routledge, 2010), 196.
11. Toulmin, "The Tyranny of Principles," 32.

12. Stephen Edelston Toulmin, *The Place of Reason in Ethics* (Cambridge: Cambridge University Press, 1970), 1.

13. Toulmin, "How Medicine Saved the Life of Ethics."

14. Edmund Pincoffs, "Quandary Ethics," *Mind* 80, no. 320 (1971): 559, italics in the original.

15. Carol Gilligan, *In a Different Voice: Psychological Theory and Women's Development*, 38th print. ed, ACLS Humanities E-Book (Cambridge, MA: Harvard University Press, 2003), 18.

16. See Nel Noddings, *Caring: A Feminine Approach to Ethics and Moral Education*, 2nd Rev. ed. (Berkeley, CA: University of California Press, 2003).

17. Alise L. Carse, "The "Voice of Care': Implications for Bioethical Education," *Journal of Medicine & Philosophy* 16, no. 1 (1991): 20.

18. Chaïm Perelman and Lucie Olbrechts-Tyteca, *The New Rhetoric: A Treatise on Argumentation* (Notre Dame, IN: University of Notre Dame Press, 1969), 444.

19. Perelman and Olbrechts-Tyteca, *The New Rhetoric: A Treatise on Argumentation*, 445.

20. Edward Schiappa, "Arguing about Definitions," *Argumentation* 7 (1993): 412.

21. Henry K. Beecher, "A Definition of Irreversible Coma: Report of the Ad Hoc Committee of the Harvard Medical School to Examine the Definition of Brain Death," *Journal of the American Medical Association* 205, no. 6 (1968): 337–340.

22. Henry K. Beecher, "After the Definition of Irreversible Coma," *New England Journal of Medicine* 281, no. 19 (1969), 947.

23. Schiappa, "Arguing about Definitions," 409.

24. James L. Bernat, Charles M. Culver, and Bernard Gert, "On the Definition and Criterion of Death," *Annals of Internal Medicine* 94, no. 3 (1981): 391.

25. Bernat, Culver, and Gert, "On the Definition and Criterion of Death," 390.

26. As quoted in Gross and Dearin, *Chaim Perelman*, 82.

27. Perelman and Olbrechts-Tyteca, *The New Rhetoric: A Treatise on Argumentation*, 412.

28. Perelman and Olbrechts-Tyteca, *The New Rhetoric: A Treatise on Argumentation*, 411.

29. Perelman and Olbrechts-Tyteca, *The New Rhetoric: A Treatise on Argumentation*, 411–412.

30. Perelman and Olbrechts-Tyteca, *The New Rhetoric: A Treatise on Argumentation*, 411.

31. Tom L Beauchamp, "The Origins and Evolution of the Belmont Report," in *Belmont Revisted*, ed. James F. Childress, Eric M. Meslin, and Harold T. Shapiro (Washington, DC: Georgetown University Press, 2005), 15.

32. Beauchamp, "The Origins and Evolution of the Belmont Report," 15–16.

33. Lainie Friedman Ross, "Health Care Decisionmaking by Children is it in their Best Interest?," *Hastings Center Report* 27, no. 6 (1997): 42.

34. See David J. Rothman, *Strangers at the Bedside: A History of How Law and Bioethics Transformed Medical Decision Making* (New York: Basic Books, 1991).

35. Mark Siegler, "Clinical Ethics and Clinical Medicine," *Archives of Internal Medicine* 139, no. 8 (1979): 914.

36. Siegler, "Clinical Ethics and Clinical Medicine," 914.
37. Siegler, "Clinical Ethics and Clinical Medicine," 914.
38. Siegler, "Clinical Ethics and Clinical Medicine," 914.
39. Siegler, "Clinical Ethics and Clinical Medicine," 915.
40. Søren Kierkegaard, *Parables of Kierkegaard*, ed. Thomas C. Oden (Princeton, NJ: Princeton University Press, 1978), 38.
41. David R. Carlin, "Rights, Animal and Human," *First Things: A Monthly Journal of Religion and Public Life* (2000) August-September, 105, 16 italics in original.
42. Carlin, "Rights, Animal and Human," 17.
43. Judith Jarvis Thomson, "A Defense of Abortion," *Philosophy and Public Affairs* 1, no. 1 (1971): 49.
44. Erik Parens, "Is Better Always Good?: The Enhancement Project," *Hastings Center Report* 28 (January–February 1998): S1–S17.
45. Parens, "Is Better Always Good?: The Enhancement Project," S1.
46. Saul A. Kripke, *Naming and Necessity* (Cambridge, MA: Harvard University Press, 1980).
47. Parens, "Is Better Always Good?: The Enhancement Project," S6.
48. Richard Huxtable and Jonathan Ives, "License to Kill: A New Model for Excusing Medically Assisted Dying?," in *New Directions in the Ethics of Assisted Suicide and Euthanasia*, ed. Michael Cholbi and Jukka Varelius (Cham: Springer, 2015), 129.
49. Willard Gaylin et al., "Doctors Must Not Kill," *Journal of the American Medical Association* 259, no. 14 (1988): 2139–2140.
50. Gaylin et al., "Doctors Must Not Kill," 2140.
51. Huxtable and Ives, "License to Kill: A New Model for Excusing Medically Assisted Dying?," 131.
52. John D. Lantos, *Do We Still Need Doctors?* (New York: Routledge, 1997), 161–162.
53. Robert Sparrow, "Defending Deaf Culture: The Case of Cochlear Implants," *Journal of Political Philosophy* 13, no. 2 (2005): 135.
54. Sparrow, "Defending Deaf Culture: The Case of Cochlear Implants," 136.
55. For example, see Michael A. Grodin and Harlan L. Lane, "Ethical Issues in Cochlear Implant Surgery: An Exploration into Disease, Disability, and the Best Interests of the Child," *Kennedy Institute of Ethics Journal* 7, no. 3 (1997): 231–251; Robert Crouch, "Let the Deaf Be Deaf: Reconsidering the Use of Cochlear Implants in Prelingually Deaf Children," *Hastings Center Report* 27, no. 4 (1997): 14–21. It should be acknowledged that these do not represent the only perspective on this issue and that one needs to recognize that alternative criticisms from disability studies, especially those that promote a social model of disability, provide a more global criticism of ableism in our society.
56. Sparrow, "Defending Deaf Culture: The Case of Cochlear Implants," 138.
57. Sparrow, "Defending Deaf Culture: The Case of Cochlear Implants," 139.
58. Gregory E. Pence, *Who's Afraid of Human Cloning?* (Lanham, MD: Rowman & Littlefield, 1998), 82.
59. Pence, *Who's Afraid of Human Cloning?*, 83.

Chapter 5

Metaphor

In the prior chapter, we examined Chaim Perelman and Lucie Olbrechts-Tyteca's concept of dissociation, through which a bioethicist is able to redescribe a concept so that what was considered a unity is shown to be two separate parts. Splitting apart something that was originally thought of as a single entity—such as the classic example in philosophy of breaking apart appearance from reality—is, however, only one direction in which arguments can be made. Its sibling concept, liaison, moves in the opposite direction, that is, bringing together elements that are not typically thought to be connected. One form of liaison explored by Perelman and Olbrechts-Tyteca is that of metaphor.

Bioethics has been particularly attentive to the role of metaphors in bioethics and medical discourse. In *The Physician's Covenant*, William May discusses how the various metaphors of the physician (e.g., fighter, technician, companion in dying) influence the manner in which we analyze moral problems in medicine.[1] Neil Manson and Onora O'Neill have observed that metaphors of conduit and container are the primary metaphors employed in discussions of informed consent.[2] Meaghan O'Keefe et al. have argued that particular metaphors dominate and in turn mediate the presentation of genetic modification to the public.[3] And Craig Klugman has analyzed the power of various metaphors used in the discussion of blood donation.[4] Indeed, the practice of bioethics itself depends upon a number of metaphors. In his criticism of the applied/theoretical distinction within moral philosophy and bioethics, Arthur Caplan takes aim at "practitioners of applied ethics [who] depict themselves as moral 'engineers' who take theoretical insights from the basic researchers and apply them to the resolution of concrete moral dilemmas."[5] Caplan assembles a healthy list of alternative metaphors for the role of the bioethicist, among them "theoretician, diagnostician, educator, coach, conceptual policeman, and skeptic."[6] In his general analysis of the role of metaphor in bioethics, James Childress adds to this list metaphors from religious categories, such as prophet and scribe,[7] and Chris MacDonald has even advocated that bioethicists embrace the metaphor of "secular priest."[8]

All of this attention to metaphor reflects a recognition of the power of metaphors to control the discourse over moral issues. Yet this recognition often focuses on metaphors like the ones above: those that characterize new technologies in terms of older technologies; those that characterize the roles of bioethicists in terms of other professions. This chapter explores other forms, such as archetypal and root metaphors, that more often go unnoticed. These metaphors also exert control over discourse—and the discourse about the proper aims and methods of bioethics is no exception.

ARCHETYPAL METAPHORS AGAINST BIOETHICS

Michael Osborn has argued that while public rhetoric may concern ephemeral issues, it tends to refer to those issues with metaphors of profound and lasting appeal, or "archetypal metaphors." As he summarizes, "Archetypal metaphors appear grounded in depth experience, such as one's susceptibility to light & darkness, one's orientation in space, family relationships, or profoundly important and vivid special experiences such as war, disease, and travel on the sea."[9] Among this category, I contend, is the spatial metaphor of inside/outside.

In describing their discipline, bioethicists often draw on physical metaphors of insider and outsider. Al Jonsen, in *The New Medicine and the Old Ethics,* discusses how he entered the field by speaking literally about entering into the medical sphere. Jonsen notes that he "eschews" carrying a beeper or donning the clinician's white coat when he shadows physicians—but still, he confesses, he feels "some gratification at being 'inside.'"[10] Perhaps to justify this feeling, Jonsen reaffirms that he has "some right to be there," for being an insider allows him to do "some good to doctors and patients."[11] In *Moral Choices*, Ruth Macklin shares the story of her own invitation to enter a hospital back in the 1970s and recalls being concerned about the reaction the physicians would have to "an outsider intruding into their domain."[12] Richard Zaner in *Troubled Voices,* describes his discomfort when he was first being consulted on ethics issues in the clinic. He characterizes his entrance into the hospital setting as his "first true adventure" and admits that initially he could not comprehend "what a person such as myself was doing there . . . inside clinical wards and units."[13] In *Bioethics as Practice*, Judith Andre characterizes the history of bioethics as a journey of outsiders, all with different reasons for making the journey to the new country of medicine.[14]

While many bioethicists allude to the pleasure and thrill of entering into the clinical world, there is also a powerful sense of dread around the prospect of becoming an insider, a danger akin to the anthropologist "going native." Later in Andre's monograph, for example, she ends her chapter on virtue in bioethics with the virtue of "being an outsider."[15] Even more overtly, Larry Churchill, in "The Ethicist in Professional Education," cautions against the bioethicist becoming "a native, a cultural insider" and relinquishing their "extraterritorial position" as an outsider to medical practice.[16] David Barnard, drawing upon Churchill's analysis, believes that bioethicists need to move on from that initial phase of entering into the sphere of medicine to one in which they imagine themselves as outsiders.[17] Here and elsewhere, the spatial metaphor of inside-outside exists as a complex proxy for how bioethicists see their relation to the clinical world. Part of the rhetoric of bioethics has been to persuade their audience that they know the world of medicine, that they are inside it—yet also, in some fundamental way, they have maintained their critical distance from that world and remain resolutely outside.

In the prior chapter, I looked at Mark Siegler's attack on bioethics, which directly addressed the spatial metaphor that has defined the discipline. Where bioethicists, many of whom were trained as moral philosophers, think their work differs from traditional moral philosophy in that it takes place inside the medical world, Siegler argues that they are not *truly* "inside." His reasoning is that being an insider is not simply being in the setting where moral problems arise, but having the responsibility for the actions taken in response to those problems. Siegler's critique only makes sense if we agree that being inside is necessary to be part of the discipline; for him, bioethicists' status as mere observers, with their "counterfeit courage of the noncombatant," are not actually inside. Yet one can also attack bioethics on the same grounds, metaphorically speaking: insiders may lack the moral distance of the outsider, rendering their judgments complicit rather than clear-eyed. One finds this basis for criticism on occasion from the social sciences, which sometimes fault bioethicists for pretending to have the moral authority of those who stand apart from the medical enterprise. In *The History and Future of Bioethics*, the sociologist John Evans' critique of bioethics extrapolates the inside-outside metaphor into other metaphors of space, ranging from practical "task spaces" and "jurisdictions" to disciplinary "expansions" and "homeland." Evans draws upon the standard sociological perspective of professions as within a level of expertise, but this expertise is viewed in terms of the governance of a particular social terrain. When discussing healthcare ethics consultations, which Evans refers to as one of bioethics' "task spaces," his metaphors are quite clear: "I am aware of no challengers for jurisdiction over this task, and I consider this to be part of the secure jurisdictional homeland of the bioethics profession."

In analogizing the field to a "watchdog," he frames this role in terms of spatial territory: "The watchdog wanders around the property, . . . If anyone intrudes, it starts to bark and growl, probably stopping the intruder."[18] And later, in his discussion of the American Society for Bioethics and Humanities' competencies, he poses the following: "Most critically, in both research bioethics and health-care ethics consultation, the watchdog must be inside the house to see any possible violations in process. But who is the master who owns the house and creates the rules?"[19] Evans' spatial metaphors reverse bioethicists' metaphors of themselves as outsiders to the medical space, allowing him to take aim at the moral assumptions that go with that characterization. Evans redescribes bioethics as simply having jurisdiction over a given social space, the role of bioethicists simply to enforce the values of the true owner of that space. Watchdogs watch over a territory; they do not own or control it.

Another key archetypal metaphor in bioethics is the vertical spatial archetype of above/below. Osborne notes that in this archetypal metaphor, our society tends to value that which is associated with above over and against those things linked to below: "Vertical scale images, which project desirable objects above the listener and undesirable objects below, often seem to express symbolically man's quest for power."[20] Interestingly, bioethics has often portrayed itself as striving to be grounded, bottom-up, and in the trenches, as opposed to moral philosophy's abstract, lofty, ivory tower perspective. Theory is most often valorized in bioethics when it is seen as closer to the ground of resolving moral problems. As John Arras notes in his discussion of the revival of casuistry in bioethics:

> In stark contrast to methods that begin "on high" with the working out of moral theory and culminate in the deductivistic application of norms to particular factual situations, this new casuistry works from the "bottom up," emphasizing practical problem-solving by means of nuanced interpretations of individual cases.[21]

In her discussion of narrative bioethics, Kathryn Montgomery argues that an attention to cases should be contrasted with theory which is "simply a 'top-down,' theory-driven activity."[22] Drew Leder argues for the superiority of a hermeneutics-informed bioethics theory over principlism by stating that the latter's "'top-down methodology,' wherein one commences with high-level theory, can obscure the rich complexity of actual cases." His proposed approach, on the other hand, is "oriented toward the close reading of narratives," allowing practitioners to "better note the significance of such elements imperceptible from the heights of ethical theory."[23] So powerful is this prioritization of the metaphorical low that Childress, in a defense of *The*

Principles of Biomedical Ethics, claims to have made a mistake by portraying the principles as literally above their specification in particular issues.[24]

Arthur Kleinman's criticism of the field demonstrates both the durability of the above/below metaphor and the same preferred orientation as Siegler and Childress. In his book *Writing at the Margin*, Kleinman often uses spatial metaphors to explain ethnographic methods in contrast to bioethics. He continually refers to how anthropological approaches to ethical issues "emerge out of the grounded experiences of sick persons," draw on "grounded perspectives," and attend to "particular local worlds." Bioethicists, in contrast, "apply the remote principles of justice and beneficence." For Kleinman, bioethics' methods "distort the practical realities among which most people on earth live,"[25] suggesting that bioethics exists in a Platonic realm apart and external to the real world, whereas anthropology, the organic and generative discipline, attends to "the cultural roots of ethical systems." Indeed, Kleinman characterizes professional bioethicists as "framing" moral issues "in high-price, high-tech, high-drama biomedical settings," reversing the tendency of bioethicists to view themselves as rooted in the practical realities of actual moral problems.

These various criticisms against bioethics are illustrative of the archetypal metaphors that have been important to bioethics. Kleinman portrays bioethics as abstract, distant, and above; Siegler sees bioethicists as not true insiders; and Evans views them as insiders who have been granted permission to guard over a particular social terrain, without any real power to govern or change that terrain. The power of these metaphor-enabled critiques resides in their ability to redescribe the archetypal metaphors that bioethics has used to characterize itself. Intriguingly, several of bioethics' metaphors of self-definition have themselves been reversals of archetypal metaphors. Height is generally viewed within Western culture as more positive than lowliness, yet bioethics has placed value on being low. Being at the center of things is generally seen from the Western vantage as better than being at the periphery, yet bioethics has prized its outsider status. Many of the metaphors used in the texts above reverse these reversals.

Archetypal metaphors have such universal power because they primarily draw upon the physical world. As Osborn has demonstrated, these metaphors have "a certain universality of appeal provided by their attachment to basic, commonly shared motives," as well, so writers who employ them "can expect such metaphors to touch the greater part of his audience."[26] In both the goal of persuasion and the effectiveness of the appeal, we see how academic disciplines might have a particular "take" on Osborn's archetypal metaphor, with the same archetypal metaphor viewed positively or negatively, depending on the particular field. Traditional moral philosophy tends to see the metaphor of up as akin to providing a superior view of a moral problem, while bioethics has tended to value instead being as close to the ground as possible (the metaphor of "down"). There is another set of metaphors in bioethics argumentation that may have even greater persuasive power than these spatial archetypes (with their susceptibility to reversal). These essential metaphors undergird *all* bioethics arguments, and as such are termed by Stephen Pepper as "root metaphors."

ROOT METAPHORS AND BIOETHICS THEORY

Pepper's notion of a root metaphor is related to a greater argument he makes concerning the existence of a number of "world hypotheses" or worldviews that underlie philosophical positions. These worldviews are derived and grounded in a particular metaphor that, in turn, directs and controls the philosophical discourse of this hypothesis:

> A man desiring to understand the world looks about for a clue to its comprehension. He pitches upon some area of commonsense fact and tries to understand other areas in terms of this one. This original area becomes his basic analogy or root metaphor. He describes as best he can the characteristics of this area, or, if you will, discriminates its structure. A list of its structural characteristics becomes his basic concepts of explanation and description. We call them a set of categories. In terms of these categories he proceeds to study all other areas of fact whether uncriticized or previously criticized. He undertakes to interpret all facts in terms of these categories. As a result of the impact of these other facts upon his categories, he may qualify and readjust the categories, so that a set of categories commonly changes and develops. Since the basic analogy or root metaphor normally (and probably at least in part necessarily) arises out of common sense, a great deal of development and refinement of a set of categories is required if they are to prove adequate for a hypothesis of unlimited scope. Some root metaphors prove more fertile than others, have greater powers of expansion and of adjustment. These survive in comparison with the others and generate the relatively adequate world theories.[27]

Pepper's concept of root metaphors is drawn upon by the cultural anthropologist Victor Turner (1974) in an examination of how metaphors influence academic thinking.[28] In explaining how academic metaphors work, Turner surveys how metaphors in general work and finds that his own understanding of metaphor is similar to I. A. Richards' "interaction view," which entails having "two thoughts of different things active together and supported by a single word, or phrase, whose meaning is a resultant of their interaction."[29] In the construction of this relationship, "The metaphor selects, emphasizes, suppresses, and organizes features of the principal subject by implying statements about it that normally apply to the subsidiary subject."[30] Seeing this process at work within the discipline of bioethics is particularly important, for it reveals the way in which root metaphors control the discipline's discourse. I hold that specific root metaphors can be found in the philosophical positions within various bioethics theories, and that the disagreement among theories is more a disagreement about the worldview behind the root metaphor than on the particular theory itself. In order to illustrate this, I look at discussions of disagreement among the various theoretical positions in bioethics and reveal that the framing of these issues occurs primarily through root metaphors, metaphors that the arguer does not share with the person who made the position with which they disagree. The description of a theory through an implicit root metaphor makes the argument persuasive to those who share the worldview that undergirds the metaphor, but the particular description will lack the power to convince those that do not already view the world through this metaphor.

ORGANICISM AND MECHANISM

In *Bioethics: A Systematic Approach* (2006), Bernard Gert, Charles M. Culver, and K. Danner Clouser provide a sustained attack on Tom Beauchamp and James Childress' (1994) theory of principlism, especially as it has been argued for in *The Principles of Biomedical Ethics*. This attack must be understood in relation to Gert, Culver, and Clouser's own proposal for a moral theory that they refer to as "common morality as a public system," which they assert "is fundamentally at odds with most of the current approaches to bioethics."[31] Close attention to the language that Gert and colleagues use, both in their critique of principlism as well as in the response to this criticism Beauchamp and Childress make, reveals that both sides are working from very different root metaphors. So while at first both sides appear to be sharing the same general approach to theory in bioethics, they do not agree in terms of their conceptual worldview and thus cannot come to terms on what is truly at stake in the disagreement.

Bioethics: A Systematic Approach is, in some ways, a profoundly intertextual product. It is the second edition of a book that had as its previous subtitle "A Return to Fundamentals." But that first edition was, in actuality, a rewritten work originally created by Culver and Gert called *Philosophy in Medicine*.[32] The revision of *Philosophy in Medicine* kept much of the discussion of particular issues within bioethics, but it also included an explicit exposition of a particular normative approach to bioethics issues and the criticism against principlism that has its source in an article by Clouser and Gert, "A Critique of Principlism," which appeared in the journal *Medicine and Philosophy* in 1990.[33]

In the 2006 version of this work, the new subtitle reveals a great deal about what is a key term for the work, systematic. Contrary to what they consider to be ad hoc judgments on moral issues, Gert, Culver, and Clouser believe that their account of philosophical justification is the only one that provides an organic connection between the moral resolutions (or why particular resolutions are not solvable) proposed and a coherent theory for those resolutions. This theory is derived from a prior common morality shared by all human beings. In making this claim, they argue, their system

> recognizes that morality is an ongoing human enterprise that long predates the attempts of any philosopher to understand it. It also means that the philosopher's systematic and explicit account of morality will be grounded in the ordinary practice of morality. This system of morality must not go against the firm and basic intuitions expressed in ordinary morality. In that sense, the philosopher "discovers" (or, perhaps, "uncovers") morality rather than invents it.[34]

This notion of "discovering" or "uncovering" a morality and developing it in relation to the ongoing public morality suggests that the root metaphor for Gert, Culver, and Clouser's work is what Pepper refers to as organicism. As the name suggests, the root metaphor for organicism is organic forms,

> the complex, integrated organic process that is presumed to underlie the development of a phenomenon, which begins in one form, then undergoes change toward some end, and finally culminates in another form that must have been implicit in the earlier form(s). Organismic philosophical systems . . . assume that the phenomena of the world exist as parts of some larger unfolding whole that is in the process of developing toward some final end state that is an integrated whole.[35]

Gert, Culver, and Clouser's tendency toward organicism is perhaps most tellingly revealed in the manner in which they criticize principlism as it is embodied in *Principles of Biomedical Medicine*, which Gert, Culver, and Clouser consider "an unsystematic and ad hoc collection of independent principles." According to Gert, Culver, and Clouser, principles, as used in principlism, are not action guides that fit within a coherent moral system but are derived from a number of different moral theories, for there are "no underlying connections among the principles. They do not grow out of a common foundation, and there is no systematic relationship among them."[36] Because the principles do not grow out of a common theoretical grounding, they are merely an eclectic and to some degree arbitrary selection of principles and, thus, not a coherent system. Gert, Culver, and Clouser are criticizing principlism for essentially not being an organic theory and for lacking the coherence they contend is necessary for any theory to be taken seriously.

As Steven Hayes and colleagues assert: "The truth criterion of organicism is coherence. When a network of interrelated facts converges on a conclusion, the coherence of this network renders this conclusion 'true.' All contradiction[s] of understanding originate in incomplete knowledge of the whole organic process."[37] The eclecticism of principlism, for Gert, Culver, and Clouser, betrays how it is not an organic whole, and through this criticism they once again reveal how organicism is the root metaphor for their understanding of normative theory and how, in turn, they evaluate moral positions that are expressions of alternative root metaphors: "The traditional concept of an ethical principle has been one that embodies the moral theory that spawns it."[38] Pepper observes that in terms of organicism, fragments of any form are antithetical to the root metaphor, for a fragment represents some element that is not integrated into the whole. In many ways, Gert, Culver, and Clouser believe that one of the central problems with principlism as a theory is that the principles themselves seem to be fragments: "there is no attempt to see how different features can be blended together as integrated parts of a single adequate theory, rather than disparate features derived from several competing theories," and so in the end we are left with moral directives that "are only superficially interrelated, having no unified, systematic, underlying foundation."[39]

Beauchamp and Childress respond in later editions of *Principles of Biomedical Ethics* to criticisms by Gert, Culver, and Clouser. Beauchamp and Childress reveal the manner in which they understand moral theory through a fundamentally different root metaphor, which is mechanistic rather than organic. According to Hayes and colleagues (1998):

> The mechanist's goal is to discover the parts and the relations among parts of the existent machine. Because mechanism is integrative, all the parts are assumed to fit together. Order is categorical. Thus, mechanists do not simply describe parts in the commonsense world; rather, they seek to discover the true nature of a given event by specifying what kind of part it really is and by placing it properly in the machine.[40]

While Gert, Culver, and Clouser wish a moral theory to grow from a common morality, Beauchamp and Childress refer to common morality as something that they "build" upon, rather than something that is discovered. For Beauchamp and Childress, theory is something that is "constructed" by the ethicist, and this position draws on the worldview of mechanism. Beauchamp and Childress list eight conditions for a "more or less traditional understanding" of the criteria one can use to judge an ethical theory. The root metaphor of the machine is expressed in a number of their criteria, such as "explanatory power," "justificatory power," "output power," and "practicality." They refer to a theory as needing to "generate," "construct," and "produce" resolutions to problems. In their discussion of "deliberation and justification," Beauchamp and Childress present, as mentioned earlier, a now often-cited and criticized model for ethics, which consists of hierarchical levels in which each level functions as a support for the other. The top tier is "ethical theories," followed by "principles," then "rules," and, at the bottom, "particular judgments and actions." This seems to represent their general approach to bioethics as a structure with each part functioning to produce more specifications in relation to particular moral quandaries.

As Franklin Berry explains:

> Mechanistic philosophical systems . . . assume that the phenomena of the world can be understood by analyzing them into their "working parts," each with a specific location, and by specifying how each part is acted on by other parts, all within a specifiable antecedent-consequent time sequence.[41]

In later editions of *The Principles of Biomedical Ethics*, Beauchamp and Childress complicate their deductivism with a discussion of inductivism and coherentism, which looks at how moral theorizing can occur bottom-up, as well as between the two. In their discussion of the coherence accounts of truth, Beauchamp and Childress express again the kind of worldview Pepper argues is part of the mechanist metaphor:

> If a stable coherence is achieved after repeated testing, the best explanation is that the system of scientific beliefs so achieved either expresses or approximates the truth. If this is a sound account of scientific truth, is it not likewise a sound account of moral truth?[42]

According to Pepper (1942), mehanists have adopted a theory of truth that is primarily operational, for which truth is determined through "the predictive power of these [sentences or formulas] to produce expected results,"[43] so that mechanists "gravitate toward" a "hypothetic-deductive research methodology."[44]

As one studies the back and forth between Gert, Culver, and Clouser and Beauchamp and Childress, one might initially conclude that the two sides differ fundamentally in terms of how they approach moral problems, but the truth is that they are far closer to each other in terms of their top-down justification, their theory of common morality, and their insistence on the importance of specification to particular problems. There is one point in Gert, Culver, and Clouser's (2006) discussion of their moral theory in which they draw upon a mechanical metaphor: "It is true that common morality is systematic enough that a computer could be programmed so that, provided with the facts of the case, it always comes up with acceptable moral answers."[45]

Yet they immediately point out this metaphor's inadequacy: "However, another computer could be programmed differently and still always come up with acceptable but different answers. There is no computer program that can tell you which of the competing computer programs you should adopt."[46] Their discussion of a computer program for moral resolution is their answer to why one needs to integrate "human judgment" into the analysis of moral problems within the common morality system, and it is in some manner an organic rebuttal to any attempt to draw upon a mechanical solution to moral problems.

FORMISM

The theoretical foundation in bioethics that has the clearest relationship to a particular worldview is casuistry, which has had its classic expression in Albert Jonsen and Stephen Toulmin's *The Abuse of Casuistry*. Casuistry is a moral theory that expresses what Pepper refers to as formism, which has as its root metaphor "similarity." Pepper argues that this worldview stems from the commonsense observation that there are similarities among the objects in our world, such as "blades of grass leaves on a tree, a set of spoons."[47] While, as Pepper notes, each of the items in these groupings is "not exactly alike," the worldview of formism attends primarily to the similarities among individual item's. An item's meaning and significance reside in being viewed as one example of a class. As Hayden White explains, the worldview behind formism "considers an explanation to be complete when a given set of objects has been properly identified, its class, generic, and specific attributes assigned, and labels attesting to its particularity attached to it."[48]

The casuist also makes comparisons among things to find similarities and constructs classes of particular cases in terms of maxims that bring them together. Jonsen breaks the casuistic method into three categories: morphology, taxonomy, and kinetics. The casuist must determine, first, the morphology of a particular case, which entails determining the case's "invariant structure." This structure, for Jonsen, represents the "deep grammar" of the case and, in turn, becomes that which is used to classify the case with other cases. After establishing the morphology of the case, the next step is taxonomy. In this step, the case is essentially classified as being a particular type. These types are established through their morphological relation to a paradigm case—that is, a case "in which the circumstances were clear, the relevant maxim unambiguous and the rebuttals weak, in the minds of almost any observer."[49] As opposed to the worldview of *contextualism*, which I discuss below, Jonsen argues that one of the key features of casuistry is that no case is unique. The final step is what Jonsen terms *kinetics*, "in which one case imparts a kind of moral movement to other cases." This construction of a taxonomy resembles the kind of thinking that goes into the natural sciences, and Jonsen is quite explicit that casuistry is a sibling discipline to the kind of work done in the biological sciences.

> the branches of physics that have cosmological ambitions . . . still refer in practice to concrete objects and situations and so are dependent on laboratory experiment and astronomical observation. The disciplines of biology lie further along the spectrum: biological theory does not aspire to abstractness or universality of physical and chemical theory: rather, biologists select a specific "subject matter" and objects of study, using taxonomic keys and other identification techniques.[50]

Understanding casuistry as a worldview with its allegiance set to a particular root metaphor helps explain the curiously harsh attack that casuists have tended to launch against principlism. Toulmin's essay "The Tyranny of Principles" seems to argue that the source of the lack of progress in ethics is the mechanistic elements of principle-based approaches in ethical theory. As mentioned in the previous chapter, he tells how during his work as a staff member with the National Commission for the Protection of Human Subjects of Biomedical and Behavioral Research, he came to realize that the disagreements were the result of discussions about abstract principles and that these disagreements never manifested themselves when they were attending to particular cases:

> So, by the end of my tenure with the Commission I had begun to suspect that the point of "appealing to principles" was something quite else: not to give particular ethical judgments a more solid foundation, but rather to square the collective ethical conclusions of the Commission as a whole with each individual commissioner's other nonethical commitments.[51]

Similarly, Toulmin blames the lack of progress on the issue of abortion in the United States on how "much of the public rhetoric increasingly came to turn on 'matters of principle'" and the way a particular problem in social welfare benefits did not require additional rules but phronesis.[52] Casuistry is, of course, his solution to these troubles.

Interestingly, in his discussion of kinetics, Jonsen clearly rejects the mechanical metaphor for this method:

> The kinetics of casuistry is not mechanical, as its counterpart in physics. One renown [*sic*] casuist was called by his modern biographer, "a marvelous moral computer," but he was an aberration, representing the decay of casuistry. Quite the contrary of mechanical or mathematical reasoning, casuistry is in essence prudential reasoning.[53]

In discussing the formist worldview, Pepper observes that it always guards itself against becoming mechanistic, and that in some manner the mechanist and the formalist are very loosely related to one another.

> The laws of nature may not be so discrete, so separate from one another, as the formist assumes. The laws of temporal and spatial structure, of gravitation, and of inertia are not now regarded as separate laws, but as the structure of a cosmic field. If all laws were amalgamated in this way into the structural skeleton of a universe, then what scientific descriptions would successively approximate would not be numbers of separate subsistent forms, but the single concrete existential structure of the universe. There would be no subsistence left. This is the mechanistic interpretation. The integration of scientific laws into a single system is thus a constant threat to the validity of formism. As long as that integration is not complete, formism has a case.[54]

So, in terms of casuistry, if one generalizes the maxims too much, one ends with principles. For those who do not see the field of bioethics as consisting of enough differentiation as that proposed by the casuists, one can see casuistry as simply a primitive stage toward the mechanical worldview of principlism.

Mark Kuczewski has argued that casuistry and principlism are similar in the manner in which they analyze moral issues. As part of his proof, he notes that Clouser and Gert's characterization of principlism is "virtually identical to casuistry."[55] Kuczewski argues that although Jonsen and Toulmin draw on the language of "maxims" or "rules of thumb," and Beauchamp and Childress on "principles," they are essentially talking about the same level of generalization and the need to apply a type of Aristotelian phronesis to resolve particular cases. Kuczewski goes on to note that "in addition to the language of mid-level principles, both casuist and principlist perceive the role of the ethicist to be one of 'weighing' or 'balancing' considerations."[56] This seems to indicate that the two approaches share a particular metaphor for understanding moral decision-making. Beauchamp and Childress (1994) do explicitly speak of this metaphor: "The metaphor of larger and smaller weights moving a scale up and down has often been invoked to depict the balancing process."[57] This self-conscious use of the scale metaphor reflects once again the manner in which the mechanist worldview informs how mechanists view moral reasoning.

One does not find a discussion of balancing (from Kuczewski's reference) in anything in *The Abuse of Casuistry*. Instead, Jonsen and Toulmin discuss the weight of an argument in casuistry as being akin to rhetoric rather than to traditional philosophical logical proofs. Jonsen does, however, explicitly discuss the notion of weight, balancing, and scales in "Casuistry as Methodology in Clinical Ethics," and it is worth quoting in full:

> Another metaphor frequently used in moral discourse speaks of reasons being "weighty" and of "balancing considers." Again, moral kinetics comes into play, since these metaphors suggest that claims can be moved up and down, from right to wrong, by adding certain "considerations" to the scale of reasoning. In reading the classical casuists, one finds that cases frequently turn on whether a sum of money is large or small, an act of aggression slight or violent, a promise about a serious or frivolous matter. The introduction of these "quantities" into moral reasoning is crucial to casuistry. On the contrary, quantifiable circumstances are rather an embarrassment to moral theory; it is very difficult to deal with "a little utility" or "a certain amount of autonomy." As we mentioned above, the weight of principles is a metaphor that is heard differently by the casuists and by the moral theorist.[58]

Jonsen is arguing that weight means very different things to a casuist than it would to a traditional moral theorist, like a principlist. His description suggests that weight is not as metaphorical for the casuist—that is, when a casuist is referring to weight, he or she is often referring to the *physical* elements of a case, elements that can be quantified. This, in turn, is not weighing on a scale, as in the weighing of moral principles, but may entail literally determining the weight of something as an aspect of the case, so the literal weight of an object can determine its place in the moral taxonomy. The taxonomy itself does not function as a scale, as a machine, but is rather a competency in judging the relevance of particularity, and in turn in comparing cases. Kuczewski's argument for bringing casuistry and principlism together may actually cause the opposite—that is, it may generate greater animosity between the two concepts. The hidden similarity between the two, which Kuczewski persuasively demonstrates, may actually be why the casuists strongly desire to maintain principlism as an adversary. Toulmin may be correct about the tyranny of principlism but not because it increases disagreement in its emphasis on abstraction; rather, there may be an unacknowledged fear that casuistry is simply a primitive stage of principlism.

CONTEXTUALISM

Zaner's *Ethics and the Clinical Encounter* typifies bioethics theory that expresses the fourth worldview Pepper discusses, contextualism. The root metaphor for contextualism is "historic event," but by this Pepper does not mean simply an event that has occurred in the past; Pepper means "the event in its actuality," in its own ongoing relation within a particular setting of time and place. This emphasis on the event entangled within a particular context thwarts any attempt to provide simple formalist generalizations, such as those seen in casuistry. Compare Pepper's characterization of contextualism with

Zaner's discussion of what he refers to as the development of a "responsive ethics." Zaner contends that a responsive ethics is the only valid and effective way to proceed in clinical ethics, for

> an ethics must become well informed about the facts of the case—not only the medical facts but other facts as well. Or, to the extent that only some facts and not others are considered (or, are at hand at the time one is asked to consider a case), the range of moral deliberations will be correspondingly limited—and so, too, for proposed moral judgments. *Moral issues are presented solely within the contexts of their actual occurrence*. Hence, it is not possible to know just which issues are actually presented by a specific case in advance of knowing the actual circumstances of their occurrence, much less to know how they might be handled or how best to propose possible resolutions in advance of having the facts well in hand.[59]

Zaner states that when we face specific cases in the clinical environment, we come "to realize that we have neither the wisdom nor a sort of moral calculus to instruct us on what any set of moral principles may or may not require of us."[60] He claims that one essentially must respond to situations only in terms of the uniqueness of that particular situation, and thus cannot come to any notion of the construction of a moral machine, prior moral categories for comparison, or some prior organic theoretical whole to resolve such issues. In describing his method, Zaner essentially outlines the various social contexts that a clinical ethicist needs in order to appropriately respond to each case, such as federal regulations, the medical institution, professional organizations, hospital policies, and the relationships among the nurses, physicians, and consultants. The ethicist does not resolve a problem by bringing a prepared system in which the problem is analyzed; instead, the ethicist is akin to an ethnographer, who must come to understand the particular case within a particular context. One cannot compare cases, as within the worldview of the formalist, for each case must not be reduced to a principle or prior category but instead must be understood solely in terms of its singular presentation.

Zaner provides three guidelines for the professional ethicist:

1. The work of ethics requires strict focus on the specific situational definition of each involved person.
2. Moral issues are present solely within the context of their actual occurrences.
3. The situational participants are the principal resources for the resolution of the moral issues presented.

Even when Zaner discusses the historical foundations of contemporary medicine or the theory of a general phenomenology, the individual event is always viewed as unique and requiring attention to its particularities, which then thwarts any attempt to submit what he views as reductionist universal principles for clinical ethics. This focus on "the specific situation," "the actual occurrence," and "the situational participants" reveals how Zaner is arguing that no universal principles or methods exist within clinical ethics. This condemnation of the permanent is, for Pepper, a key feature of the worldview expressed in contextualism. Pepper observes:

> Contextualism is constantly threatened with evidences for permanent structures in nature. It is constantly on the verge of falling back upon underlying mechanistic structures, or of resolving into the overarching implicit integrations of organicism. Its recourse in these emergencies is always to hurry back to the given event, and to emphasize the change and novelty that is immediately felt there, so that sometimes it seems to be headed for an utter skepticism. But it avoids this impasse by vigorously asserting the reality of the structure of the given event, the historic event as it actually goes on. The whole universe, it asserts, is such as this event is, whatever this is.[61]

This emphasis on the uniqueness of all moral problems can be seen in the manner that Martha Montello explicates such an approach in an essay advocating for a narrative approach to bioethics: "Always context-embedded and particular, narrative knowledge is concerned with examining and understanding singular events within the specific time and place of a unique life-story."[62] While one might argue that story in the application of narrative bioethics becomes a form that threatens to provide an organic whole, the value placed upon the contextual uniqueness of every patient's life thwarts the imposition of any closed system. This rejection of organicism within narrative ethics can be seen in Arthur Frank's typology of patient narratives, a typology that has included an anti-formalist category.[63] Frank classifies patient narratives into three types: restitution, quest, and chaos. The chaos narrative is one that seems to be a form of narrative that refuses to take on a form:

> Stories are chaotic in their absence of narrative order. Events are told as the storyteller experiences life; without sequence or discernible causality. The lack of coherent sequence is an initial reason why chaos stories are hard to hear; the teller is not understood as telling a "proper" story.[64]

As Pepper explains:

> disorder is a categorical feature of contextualism, and so radically so that it must not even exclude order. That is, the categories must be so framed as not to exclude from the world any degree of order it may be found to have, nor to deny that this order may have come out of disorder and may return into disorder

> again—order being defined any way you please, so long as it does not deny the possibility of disorder or another order in nature also.[65]

Contextualism demands that change, that fluidity, be the only thing that one cannot deny. As opposed to the Platonism of the principlist or the Aristotelianism of the casuist, contextual approaches in bioethics seem to be echoes of a Heraclitian worldview of constant change. Frank's typology that includes a critique of typology reveals the manner in which narrative ethics is in many ways the ideal illustration of the contextualist worldview.

In his general discussion of root metaphors and their worldviews, Pepper indicates that each worldview is "autonomous," and thus that one worldview cannot disprove another. Pepper also points out that each worldview is able to disparage other worldviews and to show their inadequacy:

> "You see," they say, "we are able to explain what these other mistaken philosophers have thought to be facts, and to show where the errors of their observations lay, how they rationalized their prejudices, accepting interpretations for facts and missing the real facts. Our hypothesis includes theirs and is accordingly the true account of the nature of things."[66]

Each worldview interprets the claims of the other worldviews in terms of their particular worldview. So Beauchamp and Childress are able to explain the inadequacy of Clouser, Gert, and Culver's theory through a mechanist worldview, and Clouser, Gert, and Culver can do likewise for principlism through their organicism.

There is no unbiased sphere from which one can judge the validity of the various worldviews, for it is the role of the worldview to provide a schema for judgment. For example, so enmeshed is Zaner in the contextual worldview that, in his contribution to a collection of essays on principlism, he begins with the statement:

> This essay veers away from the prevailing view in biomedical ethics: the applied, or principlist, view. Working within the clinical setting for the past decade has convinced me that it is erroneous to begin with presumptions, even the presumptions that physicians are supposed to be governed by beneficence and patients by autonomy. . . . It is nonetheless perhaps more productive to probe these encounters in more depth than has been usual, before making up one's mind about such austere matters as ethical principles.[67]

Zaner's contextualism is his presumption against all presumptions. Similarly, Toulmin, in his argument against the tyranny of principles, begins by seeing that the appeals to "matters of principles" are in reality appeals to "narrow dogmatism," and such appeals are, within his particular worldview, an expression of problems with our moral discourse, not a way to resolve our problems.

What is at stake in uncovering the various metaphors within the debates over theory in bioethics? Pepper's linking of the metaphorical roots of philosophical positions to particular worldviews challenges the provenance of disagreements in academic discourse. That is, our disagreements have less to do with conscious rational choices that we make when we argue for the superiority of a particular theory than they do with expressions of a worldview that we possess prior to the theory. Thus, what has come to be termed in bioethics the "theory wars" may perhaps be better called the "root metaphor wars," and an understanding of the poetics of metaphor can be seen to be crucial to understanding how theory is done in bioethics.

CONCLUSION

Most analyses of metaphor in bioethics have been on the explicit, or at least the not-particularly-hidden, metaphors within the field's discourse. This chapter has focused on metaphors that, in many ways are less evident than those usually studied, such as the engineering or priestly metaphors mentioned at the start of this chapter. While archetypal and root metaphors are not as easily perceived as more explicit ones, their influence can be said to be more profound, for they direct an argument through evocation. As Sonja Foss observes, "[m]etaphor does not simply provide support for an argument; instead, the structure of the metaphor itself argues."[68] In terms of Pepper's typology, our description of the world through a particular root metaphor can mean the acceptance or rejection of an argument even before the argument has taken place, depending on whether or not we share the worldview embedded in the root metaphor guiding the analysis. This chapter has focused on metaphors, and the next chapter will look at how metaphor is a form of analogy and thus an expression of thinking through similitude. For the rhetorician Richard Weaver, similitude is just one "source" for an argument. The next chapter examines the ways other sources for arguments are used in bioethics.

NOTES

1. William F. May, *The Physician's Covenant: Images of the Healer in Medical Ethics*, 2nd ed. (Lexington, KY: Westminster John Knox Press, 2000).
2. Neil C. Manson and Onora O'Neill, *Rethinking Informed Consent in Bioethics* (Cambridge: Cambridge University Press, 2007).

3. Meaghan O'Keefe et al., "'Editing' Genes: A Case Study About How Language Matters in Bioethics," *The American Journal of Bioethics* 15, no. 12 (2015): 3–10.

4. Craig M. Klugman, "Blood Donation and Its Metaphors," *The American Journal of Bioethics* 10, no. 2 (2010): 46–47.

5. Arthur L. Caplan, "Ethical Engineers Need Not Apply: The State of Applied Ethics Today," *Science, Technology & Human Values* 5, no. 4 (1980): 26.

6. Caplan, "Ethical Engineers Need Not Apply: The State of Applied Ethics Today," 30.

7. James F. Childress, *Practical Reasoning in Bioethics*, Medical Ethics Series (Bloomington, IN: Indiana University Press, 1997).

8. Chris MacDonald, "Will the "Secular Priests" of Bioethics Work Among the Sinners?," *American Journal of Bioethics* 3, no. 2 (2003).

9. Michael Osborn, "The Trajectory of My Work with Metaphor," *Southern Communication Journal* 74, no. 1 (2009): 81.

10. Albert R. Jonsen, *The New Medicine and the Old Ethics* (Cambridge, MA: Harvard University Press, 1990), 2.

11. Jonsen, *The New Medicine and the Old Ethics*, 2.

12. Ruth Macklin, *Mortal Choices: Bioethics in Today's World* (New York: Pantheon Books, 1987), 14.

13. Richard M. Zaner, *Troubled Voices: Stories of Ethics and Illness* (Cleveland, OH: Pilgrim Press, 1993), 1–2.

14. Judith Andre, *Bioethics as Practice* (Chapel Hill, NC: University of North Carolina Press, 2002), 26–41.

15. Andre, *Bioethics as Practice*, 132–133.

16. Larry R. Churchill, "The Ethicist in Professional Education," *Hastings Center Report* 8 (1978): 15.

17. David Barnard, "Reflections of a Reluctant Clinical Ethicist: Ethics Consultation and the Collapse of Critical Distance," *Theoretical Medicine* 13 (1992): 15–22.

18. John Hyde Evans, *The History and Future of Bioethics: A Sociological View* (New York: Oxford University Press, 2012), 102.

19. Evans, *The History and Future of Bioethics: A Sociological View*, 102.

20. Michael Osborn, "Archetypal Metaphor in Rhetoric: The Light-Dark Family," *Quarterly Journal of Speech* 53, no. 2 (1967): 116.

21. John D. Arras, "Getting Down to Cases: The Revival of Casuistry in Bioethics," *The Journal of Medicine and Philosophy*, no. 1 (February 1991): 30.

22. Kathryn Montgomery Hunter, "Narrative," in *Encyclopedia of Bioethics*, ed. Warren T. Reich (New York: Simon & Schuster, 1995), 1791.

23. Drew Leder, "Toward a Hermeneutical Bioethics," in *A Matter of Principles?: Ferment in U.S. Bioethics*, ed. E. R. DuBose, R. P. Hamel, and L. J. O'Connel (Valley Forge, PA: Trinity, 1994), 251.

24. James Childress, "Principles-Oriented Bioethics: An Analysis and Assessment from Within," in *A Matter of Principles?: Ferment in U.S. Bioethics*, ed. Edwin R. DuBose, Ronald P. Hamel, and Laurence J. O'Connell (Valley Forge, PA: Trinity Press International, 1994), 81.

25. Arthur Kleinman, *Writing at the Margin: Discourse Between Anthropology and Medicine* (Berkeley, CA: University of California Press, 1995), 408.

26. Osborn, "Archetypal Metaphor in Rhetoric: The Light-Dark Family," 116.

27. Stephen C. Pepper, *World Hypotheses, a Study in Evidence* (Berkeley and Los Angeles, CA: University of California Press, 1942), 89–90.

28. Victor Witter Turner, *Dramas, Fields, and Metaphors; Symbolic Action in Human Society* (Ithaca, NY: Cornell University Press, 1974).

29. I. A. Richards, *The Philosophy of Rhetoric* (London: Oxford University Press, 1965), 93.

30. Turner, *Dramas, Fields, and Metaphors; Symbolic Action in Human Society*, 30.

31. Bernard Gert, Charles M. Culver, and K. Danner Clouser, *Bioethics: A Systematic Approach*, second ed. (New York: Oxford University Press, 2006), v.

32. Charles M. Culver and Bernard Gert, *Philosophy in Medicine: Conceptual and Ethical Issues in Medicine and Psychiatry* (New York: Oxford University Press, 1982).

33. K. Danner Clouser and Bernard Gert, "A Critique of Principlism," *Journal of Medicine and Philosophy* 15, no. 2 (1990): 219–236.

34. Gert, Culver, and Clouser, *Bioethics: A Systematic Approach*, 10.

35. Franklin M. Berry, "An Introduction to Stephen C. Pepper's Philosophical System via World Hypotheses: A Study in Evidence," *Bulletin of the Psychonomic Society* 22, no. 5 (1984): 448.

36. Gert, Culver, and Clouser, *Bioethics: A Systematic Approach*, 110.

37. Steven C. Hayes, Linda J. Hayes, and Hayne W. Reese, "Finding the Philosophical Core: A Review of Stephen C. Pepper's World Hypotheses: A Study in Evidence," *Journal of the Experimental Analysis of Behavior* 50, no. 1 (1988): 100.

38. Gert, Culver, and Clouser, *Bioethics: A Systematic Approach*, 99.

39. Gert, Culver, and Clouser, *Bioethics: A Systematic Approach*, 124.

40. Hayes, Hayes, and Reese, "Finding the Philosophical Core: A Review of Stephen C. Pepper's World Hypotheses: A Study in Evidence," 99.

41. Berry, "An Introduction to Stephen C. Pepper's Philosophical System via World Hypotheses: A Study in Evidence," 448.

42. Tom L. Beauchamp and James F. Childress, *Principles of Biomedical Ethics*, 4th ed. (New York: Oxford University Press, 1994), 27.

43. Pepper, *World Hypotheses, a Study in Evidence*, 255.

44. Hayes, Hayes, and Reese, "Finding the Philosophical Core: A Review of Stephen C. Pepper's World Hypotheses: A Study in Evidence," 107.

45. Gert, Culver, and Clouser, *Bioethics: A Systematic Approach*, 107.

46. Gert, Culver, and Clouser, *Bioethics: A Systematic Approach*, 107.

47. Pepper, *World Hypotheses, a Study in Evidence*, 151.

48. Hayden V. White, *Metahistory: The Historical Imagination in Nineteenth-Century Europe* (Baltimore, MD: Johns Hopkins University Press, 1973), 14.

49. Arras, "Getting Down to Cases: The Revival of Casuistry in Bioethics," 301.

50. Albert R. Jonsen, "Casuistry as Methodology in Clinical Ethics," *Theoretical Medicine* , no. 4 (1991): 36.

51. Stephen Toulmin, "The Tyranny of Principles," *Hastings Center Report* 11, no. 6 (1981): 32.

52. Toulmin, "The Tyranny of Principles," 32.

53. Jonsen, "Casuistry as Methodology in Clinical Ethics," 303.

54. Pepper, *World Hypotheses, a Study in Evidence*, 184.

55. Mark Kuczewski, "Casuistry and Principlism: The Convergence of Method in Biomedical Ethics," *Theoretical Medicine and Bioethics* 19, no. 6 (1998): 517.

56. Kuczewski, "Casuistry and Principlism: The Convergence of Method in Biomedical Ethics," 516.

57. Tom L. Beauchamp, *Principles of Biomedical Ethics*, 4th ed. (Oxford: Oxford University Press, 1994), 33.

58. Jonsen, "Casuistry as Methodology in Clinical Ethics," 304.

59. Richard M. Zaner, *Ethics and the Clinical Encounter* (Englewood Cliffs, NJ: Prentice Hall College Div, 1988), 27.

60. Zaner, *Ethics and the Clinical Encounter,* 27.

61. Pepper, *World Hypotheses, a Study in Evidence*, 234–244.

62. Martha Montello, "Narrative Competence," in *Stories and Their Limits: Narrative Approaches to Bioethics*, ed. Hilde Lindemann Nelson (London: Routledge, 1997), 190.

63. Arthur W. Frank, *The Wounded Storyteller: Body, Illness, and Ethics* (Chicago, IL: University of Chicago Press, 1995).

64. Frank, *The Wounded Storyteller: Body, Illness, and Ethics*, 97.

65. Pepper, *World Hypotheses, a Study in Evidence*, 234.

66. Pepper, *World Hypotheses, a Study in Evidence*, 99–100.

67. Richard M. Zaner, "Experience and Moral Life: A Phenomenological Approach to Bioethics," in *A Matter of Principles?: Ferment in U.S. Bioethics*, ed. E. R. DuBose, R. P. Hamel, and L. J. O'Connel (Valley Forge, PA: Trinity, 1994), 211.

68. Sonja K. Foss, *Rhetorical Criticism: Exploration and Practice*, 5th ed. (Long Grove, IL: Waveland Press, 2018), 288.

Chapter 6

Sources

In the prior chapter, we examined the way metaphors function within the discourse of bioethics. As mentioned at the beginning of that chapter, as opposed to dissociation, metaphors for Chaim Perelman and Lucie Olbrechts-Tyteca represent a form of liaison, bringing together two elements that had not before been thought to have a direct connection. Perelman and Olbrechts-Tyteca consider metaphor a subset of the process of analogical thinking, which has long been recognized as a central feature of bioethics arguments.[1] Its centrality is most obvious in casuistry, for the construction of a typology based on similarities to a paradigm case is clearly a form of thinking based upon analogical formulations. Indeed, Albert Jonsen and Stephen Toulmin define casuistry as the interpretation of moral problems "using procedures of reasoning based on paradigms and analogies."[2] James Childress argues that analogy is fundamental not merely to casuistry but to ethics in general, as it manifests our shared assumption that there is a "moral requirement to treat similar cases in a similar way."[3] Analogical reasoning is not without its critics in bioethics, especially in cases where readers are asked to accept a new practice or novel technology on the basis of its similarity to a prior practice or technology. In such instances, one might perceive a necessarily conservative quality of analogical thinking, in that anything shown to be comparable to existing practices should automatically be allowed.

In "Abortion and Argument by Analogy," Lisa Sowle Cahill identifies a number of ways analogical thinking in bioethics can lead to the misrepresentation or neglect of essential features of an argument. In the prior chapter on dissociation, one example analyzed was Judith Jarvis Thomson's "unconscious violinist" thought experiment, in which a violinist is "plugged in" to a non-consenting person for a period of time in order to keep the musician alive. This thought experiment permits Thomson to reorient the bioethical debate from the status of the fetus's personhood to the contentious obligation to keep *any* other person alive, if doing so deprives someone of their liberty. While acknowledging that such analogies assist us in thinking through the moral dimensions of the abortion debate, Cahill sees a serious flaw in Thomson's thought experiment, which "places the offspring in the role of an alien being"[4] and thus does not attend to the unique ontology of human pregnancy—that is, something without analogy.

A key rhetorical move of Peter Singer's book *Animal Liberation*, in addition to his vivid redescriptions of meat-making and eating, is the analogy he draws between speciesism, racism, and sexism. As he points out, arguments based on intellect, such as specious arguments claiming the superiority of one race or gender over another, should not be credited: even if they are proven true by some measure, one's worth as a person of equal value to others does not reside in one's intellectual abilities.

> It is on this basis that the case against racism and the case against sexism must both ultimately rest; and it is in accordance with this principle that the attitude that we may call "speciesism," by analogy with racism, must also be condemned. . . . It should be obvious that the fundamental objects to racism and sexism . . . apply equally to speciesism. If possessing a higher degree of intelligence does not entitle one human to use another for his or her own ends, how can it entitle humans to exploit nonhumans for the same purpose?[5]

The terms "racism" and "sexism" are, for our society, what the rhetorician Richard Weaver refers to as "devil terms." As opposed to a "god term," "devil terms" define that which a society finds to be ultimately "repulsive";[6] at the time of the term's coinage, Weaver gave as examples such words as "Communism" and "un-American." Singer, by creating an analogous relationship between racism/sexism and the belief that the human species is fundamentally different and superior to other species, makes a devil term of speciesism. Yet the belief that humans are qualitatively different from all other animals, and that this difference allows humans to act upon non-human animals in a manner that would not be permitted on other humans, is actually one that has been traditionally held in almost all societies. Once we acknowledge this broader context, we can see that speciesism is not universally accepted as a devil term. Still, in creating this analogy, Singer is able to portray this orientation as an insidious prejudice against other species, another instance of a well-known and spurious belief.

Another important concept in rhetorical analysis developed by Weaver was his notion of attending to the sources of an argument. Weaver argues that certain sources distill and express the author's worldview, constituting "the persuasive foundation—the strategic center—of an argument."[7] Acknowledging that there will be a number of sources for justification in any lengthy argument, Weaver observes that there tends to be a "predominating [or focal] source" which resides in the major premise of the argument. It is within this argument that the focal source is revealed, and it is this focal source that reveals the character of the arguer. Weaver contends that no person "escapes being branded by the premise" they think is most valuable to promote.[8] In short, Weaver asserts, the method used in an argument is a "truer index" of a person's beliefs than any "explicit profession of principles."[9]

To investigate that method, Weaver created a typology of sources that "invokes essential correspondences and includes analogy, metaphor, figuration, comparison, and contrast."[10] Weaver held that arguments based on similitude, like analogical thinking, reflected an author who "tend[s] to look toward some final transcendental unity."[11] This description is an apt one for Singer, whose wish to apply the same measure to all living entities, and perception of bias in any attempt to differentiate humans from other animals, indicates his universalism. A similar worldview can be discerned in the work of Jonsen and Toulmin on behalf of casuistry. In liberating us from what they see as the cause of moral and decision-making disunity (namely, principlism), they argue, casuistry offers the promise of perfect agreement; attending to particular cases and the maxims that link those cases to other cases creates a ground for consensus that the brittle tyranny of principles never could. Perhaps paradoxically, then, analogical thinking is what creates a transcendent unity for Jonsen and Toulmin, while overarching principles actually seem to reveal disunity. In his critique of their argument for a secular casuistry, Kevin Wm. Wildes casts Jonsen and Toulmin's confidence in this unity as naïve idealism. The unity the original form of casuistry enjoyed owed entirely to its grounding in a larger moral vision within the Catholic Church, according to Wildes.[12] He faults Jonsen and Toulmin for not taking seriously the pluralism that would naturally threaten the common morality they anticipate leading to universal agreement on paradigmatic cases.

Similitude is just one form of source an arguer could draw upon. Weaver's taxonomy also included (depending on where he was in his career) genus, consequences, circumstances, history, and authority as operative sources in contemporary arguments.[13] When any of these sources became the predominant source of an argument, Weaver held, it expressed a fundamental feature of the writer's worldview. Here the contentious nature of Weaver's typology should be noted, for it was not simply descriptive but also prescriptive; Weaver believed that certain sources were more ethical than others. Weaver did not merely provide a typology of sources but also argued that the sources should be ranked ethically. At the top of his hierarchy was genus, which he contended was the most ethical form of argumentation as it represented an appeal to eternal ideals. Similitude was next, for while it did not entail a direct appeal to eternal forms, it was still based on a comparison to these forms. Next lower down were appeals to consequences, which Weaver argued were "completely devoid of reference to principle or defined ideas."[14] The bottom of Weaver's typology is an argument that is justified by way of circumstances.

Controversially, Weaver argued that political ideologies gravitated toward particular sources. He saw conservatives as tending to appeal to genus and definition, while liberals tended to appeal to circumstances. Since Weaver was an outspoken political conservative, the fact that he linked conservative arguments to genus also meant that conservatives, for him drew upon the most ethical form of argumentation. A few qualifications should be made to this depiction of his ranking, however. First, Weaver did not argue that taking a conservative view meant that one *always* drew upon genus. One notable exception in this regard was the English conservative Edmund Burke's appeal to circumstances in his analysis of the French Revolution (which Weaver found extremely objectionable).[15] Second, Weaver's concept of *liberal* was "confusing," as John Bliese remarks, in that what he meant by liberal was not a "political liberal" but rather a political position that was the "center"—and could also be interpreted to mean "relativist." Such a position indicated that one took a position between the extremes and thus one did not argue from any particular ideology but only in relation to the conditions of the moment. He saw the radical left as most often arguing from consequences, not circumstances;[16] this source, however, is still relatively low on Weaver's axiology, which was clearly constructed to support his bias toward Platonism and conservatism.

I believe that Weaver's typology can, however, be useful if one strips it of its axiological judgments. What is of interest here is the way in which arguments are framed in relation to particular sources, as well as how certain sources, such as similitude, represent a particular worldview that the reader must submit to in order to be persuaded by the argument. As Sonja Foss, Karen Foss, and Robert Trapp observe,

> when speakers use particular arguments, they are asking their listeners not simply to follow a valid reasoning form but to agree with the particular view of reality being presented. Through the use of certain argumentative sources, rhetors say that they believe in and urge acceptance of a particular construction of the universe. They seek to persuade the audience to read the world as they do.[17]

In what follows, we will look at the presence of differing sources in bioethicists' arguments and discuss the sources' relationship to the position being taken.

AUTHORITY AND TESTIMONY

Weaver differentiated arguments based on *authority*, as well as those based on the source of *testimony*, as being "external," in contrast to the sources he saw as "internal." As Weaver explains:

> The difference to be noted is that whereas the internal source, such as genus or cause, is a direct perception by us of an aspect of phenomena, the external source is a report of such perception on the part of someone else.[18]

For Weaver, to rely on testimony is to draw upon the internal worldview and contention of another person; these are arguments that are "imported from outside."[19] Similarly, arguments based on authority rely on "some other exalted source whose word on the subject in question is regarded as final."[20]

At the beginning of this book, I contrasted the world-building of Joseph Fletcher with that of Paul Ramsey. As I noted, the two men came from similar Christian faith traditions, and while they differed radically on what they argued, the source for their arguments was the same: not human rights, utilitarianism, pragmatism, or deontology—but scripture. In *Reading the Bible in the Strange World of Medicine*, Allen Verhey observes that both these Christian thinkers had a notion of persons that was based on appeals to the Bible. In *Morals and Medicine*, Fletcher draws upon the biblical notion of "the image of God" in his definition of personhood;[21] in *The Patient as Person*, Paul Ramsey draws on the biblical notion of "flesh" for his.[22] Though their interpretations diverge, both use passages from the Bible to argue for their preferred concept of a person. Verhey's discussion of these two figures from the early history of bioethics is important because the central goal of his book is to advocate for a form of the discipline whose justification lies in Christian scripture; he argues that a proper Christian bioethics should have as its guide "To search the Scriptures and to attend to God in the context of bioethics."[23]

As an illustration, in his chapter "Mapping the Human Genome . . . Biblically," Verhey first surveys the ways the human genome has been "mapped" through "genetic reductionism," Baconism, a liberal society, a quest for "perfect children," and capitalism. Verhey then proposes an alternative map based on the biblical narratives of God's creation of the world, sin, covenant, and Jesus. (I do not wish to suggest that Verhey finds a simple list of action guides in the Bible that he advises us to apply to real-world bioethical dilemmas; he is well aware that examining bioethics through Christian scripture requires interpretation, that it takes intellectual work to connect the "strange" world of contemporary medicine with the "strange" world of scripture.) Notably, Verhey does not seek to justify his alternative map for genomics beyond his appeal to scripture—a seemingly odd choice, if his audience comprises moral philosophers and secular casuists. Yet in her review of Verhey's book for the *Journal of the Catholic Health Association of the United States*, Eloise Rosenblatt points out that Verhey's book is *not* aimed "at academics, who are philosophical ethicists, but rather at the broader community—pastors and health-care professionals who seek bridges between the world of faith and the reality of the laboratory."[24] Noting the intended audience of Verhey's book helps us recognize that Verhey's appeal to the authority of the Bible is, in fact, persuasive—though only to those who already accept the Bible as persuasive. As Weaver explains,

> If a proposition is backed by some weighty authority, like the Bible, or can be associated with a great name, people may be expected to respond to it in accordance with the veneration they have for these sources. In this way, evidence coming from the outside is used to influence attitudes or conduct.[25]

Some have argued that theological voices became less prominent in bioethics when they departed from the appeal we see Verhey making. Opting not to cite the very ground of their authority—scripture—when addressing the general public, including those outside their faith tradition, their arguments were difficult to distinguish from those made by secular moral philosophers. In the end, Leon Kass has noted, this resulted in theologians sounding "just like everybody else."[26]

Similar to the source of authority, Weaver contended that an argument based on *testimony* relies "upon the credit of someone who is testifying" and thus, unlike arguments with an internal logic, its justification is external to the person actually making the argument. "By this means, statements by people presumed to be in a position to know are brought into an argument and take the place of direct or logical interpretation of evidence"; when an argument is based on this source, it is not "affirming a fact or relationship" itself, but instead affirming "that someone else affirms it."[27] Weaver's examples of how testimony functions as a source of argument are drawn almost exclusively from its use in criminal trials. For, understandably, one's innocence, even against the physical evidence, can be argued for by providing witness testimony that the accused could not have committed the crime because the witness was with the accused when the crime occurred.[28] In bioethics, the use of testimony as the source of an argument can be found in Arthur Frank's *The Wounded Storyteller*, in the notion of a postmodern ethic. The seventh chapter of his book is actually titled "Testimony," and explains that for the "wounded storytellers" to provide testimony represents a moral duty, a duty both to tell and to hear. Frank advocates that people who are in what he refers to as the "remission society" should identify themselves as "witnesses," which he prefers to the term *survivor* because survivor "does not include any particular responsibility other than continuing to survive."[29] The witness does not simply exist but has a responsibility to act, and that action for Frank is the utterance of testimony: "People who tell stories of illness are witnesses, turning illness into moral responsibility."[30] According to Frank, postmodernism has a special "affinity" for testimony as a source of argument, and the emphasis on testimony within bioethics is an expression of what Frank considers "narrative ethics." Frank views narrative ethics as based on the notion that we should "think with stories." Still, as with authority, testimony relies on the acceptance of the truth of another's experience.

John Arras has critiqued the use of testimony as a source of argument within bioethics due to the self-justifying nature of personal stories, warning that personal testimony "risks undercutting our ability to make moral judgments."[31] Howard Brody and Tom Tomlinson, respectively, have acknowledged the great value testimony has had in terms of activism for marginalized groups[32] and the political arena.[33] But Brody also includes a content note citing a misuse of testimony, when personal stories were used successfully to persuade policymakers that women with breast cancer should undergo treatment that included bone marrow transplants—a treatment that evidence-based research ended up showing to be ineffective.[34] And Tomlinson insists that testimony cannot justify moral principles, for the argument itself must be justified in the end by an appeal to principles. Thus, for Tomlinson, an appeal must be made to a source outside of the testimony.[35]

GENUS AND DEFINITION

This chapter began by identifying the appeal to similitude in Singer's argument that humans owe a particular set of moral obligations to other nonhuman animals: we should be as opposed to speciesism as we are to sexism and racism. While Singer does not base his arguments upon a notion of rights, as discussed in the chapter on anagnorisis, the argument that animals have rights has been taken up by others, most notably Tom Regan.[36] In his argument against Regan's position that animals have rights, Carl Cohen opens by targeting another argument in the "abolitionist family" based on similitude. He recalls how animal rights advocates portray the use of animals for experimentation as akin to the use of Jews by the Nazis in their hypothermia experiments, and thus the results of animal experiments should be equally condemned. So, as Cohen ventriloquizes, experimentation on animals undertaken "to immunize humans against or treat diseases such as polio, malaria, and AIDS is as profoundly wrong, as plainly *unjust*, as what was done by Nazis to those Jews not so very long ago." Then he interjects in his own voice:

> This is for them [the animal rights advocates] hyperbole. Animal rights advocates need not hold (and generally do not hold) that contemporary medical scientists are as vicious as the Nazis were. They simply believe that in the same way that what the Nazis did was morally unacceptable, what is being done to animals is not morally unacceptable.[37]

Here Cohen seems to accept the appeal to similitude, yet argues that its entailments do not hold: if animals have the rights we assume humans to have, then the analogy would not be hyperbole, but rather plain description. The term for Cohen's source here, according to Weaver's typology, is that of *genus*.

Being "based on the nature of the thing which is said to constitute its genus,"[38] arguments with genus as their source rely upon that entity having a known essence. These arguments depend on the belief that there are classes of things "which are determinate and therefore predictable."[39] From Weaver's perspective, Cohen's move from similitude to genus is quite logical, for analogical arguments get their warrant by their connection to a genus. The genus that Cohen is concerned with is that of "rights," and whether specific obligations to animals follow if we classify them as a category of being that possesses rights in the same way that humans possess them. Before exploring this, Cohen provides the definition of rights as follows: "A *right* is a valid claim, or potential claim that may be made by a moral agent under principles that govern both the claimant and the target of the claim."[40] After this definition, Cohen provides a footnote stating that this definition "expresses what most philosophers [including Tom Regan] agree is essential"[41] to the notion of rights. This note is important because Cohen is not making an argument based on definition (which we will discuss later), but on genus. Cohen's argument relies on the genus of rights already existing and being accepted by those in the discipline; he is not providing a novel argument on the nature of rights. Once Cohen establishes what a right is, he is able to argue against the Nazi analogy, for animals cannot fit within the genus of an entity that has rights:

> Animals cannot be bearers of rights because the concept of right is *essentially human*; it is rooted in the human world and has force and applicability only within that world. . . . To say of a pig or a rabbit that it has rights is to confuse categories, to apply to its world a moral category that can have content only in the human moral world.[42]

It is notable that in this quote, Cohen refers to an animal as an "it" rather than using a personal pronoun. For him, rights exist as a Platonic category that can only encompass entities that have personal pronouns. According to Weaver, arguments that use genus as their source indicate the worldview of an idealist: "the idea of genus is a reflection of existence."[43] For Cohen, the fact that animals cannot have rights is an expression of the essential reality of the world. As noted above, for Weaver, arguments such as Cohen's represent the most "ethical" form of argumentation because their appeal is to unchanging essences. In this light, one cannot argue that animals have rights any more than one can change the very nature of reality.

While Cohen's argument against animal liberation draws on a previously accepted genus (that of rights), Weaver also identified arguments whose primary aim is to define a genus. The difference between an argument whose source is definition and another whose source is genus is whether the argument itself is for a particular definition. In a genus-based argument like Cohen's, the "classification is already established"; if the source is definition, "the work of establishing the classification must be done in the course of the argument, after which the defined term will be used as would any genus."[44] Weaver contends, however, that the argument from definition still relies on the belief that "there exists classes which are determinate and therefore predictable."[45] In the end, the selection of a particular definition is, as David Zarefsky notes, "to plead a cause, as if one were advancing a claim and offering support for it."[46]

A good contrast in the bioethics of argument from genus versus one from definition can be seen in how the concept of nature is used by Leon Kass and how it is used by Gregory Kaebnick. In *Toward a More Natural Science*, Kass assumes that nature exists as an accepted genus and thus does not require him to provide an argument for a definition. As Kass himself admits in the preface to his book: "'Natural' and 'more natural' mean here only 'true' (or 'truer') to life as found and lived."[47] He goes on to claim that his use of nature in the monograph does not "imply" any particular theory or school of thought. Yet he uses the term throughout as if it simply exists as a genus, clear to all, and he bases upon it his evaluation of contemporary medical concepts and interventions. Kaebnick's book *Humans in Nature*, by contrast, is a sustained examination of nature as a genus and, to some degree an analysis of how this genus, if it can be clearly defined, is a crucial part of bioethics as a discipline.[48]

This latter form of argument is illustrated in the work of Lawrence Schneiderman and Nancy Jecker, prominent voices in the debate on the use of futility in clinical decisions. The majority of the first chapter of their book *Wrong Medicine* consists of the authors "presenting and defining a definition of futility"[49]—and that definition is in many ways the overall purpose of the book. Not "simply a description or example of futility" but an explicit definition, one their readers watch them construct, is what they seek to establish. Their rationale is that this act of definition might "provide the necessary and sufficient conditions for a medical intervention falling under the term."[50]

The construction of this genus is not a descriptive exercise for Schneiderman and Jecker but a prescriptive one. This goal is also visible in their book's structure. The first part contains their argument for their definition of futility, while the second part stages, as Thaddeus Mason Pope observes in a review, "an extended argument urging the adoption and implementation of" this definition.[51] This intellectual partisanship aligns well with Weaver's typology; he contends that definitions should not be based on empirical evidence but rather on rationality, for a definition "should be stipulative, emphasizing what ought to be, rather than operational, emphasizing what is."[52] Schneiderman and Jecker embody Weaver's ideal when they contrast their argument for a definition of medical futility against a definition from science, such as that for energy or mass. They also openly acknowledge that their definition relies upon a consensus of the values of society, pointing to the development of the brain death definition—based less on an empirical finding and more on our "society's sense of the meaning of human life"[53]—as a model.

In the course of their argument, Schneiderman and Jecker consider other definitions, including what is often referred to as the strict or physiological definition of futility. This definition holds that if a medical intervention is functioning, then the intervention is not futile. Schneiderman and Jecker object to such a definition because it does not take into account issues of quality of life and the final goals of medical care, which they contend is not simply to keep a human body alive. They then turn to another definition of futility, this one derived from the express point of view of the patient. While such a definition would certainly express respect for patient autonomy, it would also allow patients to demand any type of intervention they wanted, even if the physician believed it to be harmful or useless. Schneiderman and Jecker also reject a definition of futility that encompasses interventions that cause more harm than benefit (in addition to interventions that provide no benefit whatsoever). This definition fails on the basis of social values, they argue, for it would reclassify as futile many interventions that most would find permissible. After criticizing these prior definitions, Schneiderman and Jecker propose their own:

> Medical futility means any effort to provide a benefit to a patient that is highly likely to fail and whose rare exceptions cannot be systematically produced. Note first that this definition includes a quantitative component ("highly likely to fail") and a qualitative component ("benefit to the patient").[54]

The quantitative component entails a "practical definition" by which an intervention would be considered futile if it had not had success in the last one hundred cases. The qualitative component, for Schneiderman and Jecker, means that a treatment would be classified as futile if the patient does not possess "the capacity to appreciate the benefit of a treatment, or if the treatment fails to release a patient from total dependence on the acute hospital setting for survival."[55] Throughout this chapter, Schneiderman and Jecker are simultaneously refuting prior definitions and promoting their new definition of medical futility; in doing so, they are attempting to establish futility as a particular genus.

Finally, before leaving arguments based on genus, I would like to note the number of bioethicists who have attempted to argue from an anti-idealistic perspective. Their arguments comprise what might be called anti-genus arguments within the discipline. One instance has already been discussed in the chapter on dissociation: the Deaf community's response to cochlear implants involves a rejection of the genus of disabled, possibly prompting a larger reconsideration of the classification of disability itself. In *Leaky Bodies and Boundaries*, Margrit Shildrick promotes a postmodern feminist bioethics that has, as one of its primary focuses, an attack on the universal genus of gender.[56] And Richard Twine has argued for the deconstruction of the culture/nature dualism within the discipline.[57]

CONSEQUENCES

In the chapter on dissociation, we looked at the way Gregory Pence counters opponents of cloning (like Kass) in order to present cloning as a permissible form of reproduction. The second time Pence cites Kass is in a chapter titled "The False Seers of Assisted Human Reproduction." Pence dismisses Kass's ominous warning to the National Bioethics Advisory Commission (NBAC) in the late 1990s concerning the dangers of cloning humans by recounting how Kass had argued against IVF in the 1970s with similar concerns about the potential dangers to the children reproduced in this manner. As Pence asks,

> Why should we trust the claims to wisdom of such people? Have they ever admitted they were wrong to oppose the creation of thousands upon thousands of babies created by IVF That they misjudged the risk of harm to these babies? Are not the same premises still operative in their thinking that they assumed two decades ago, leading them now to similarly unsound conclusions?[58]

Here Pence is attacking the use of *consequences*[59] as a source for the argument against human cloning. Pence would likely agree with Weaver's dismissal of arguments based on this source as "sensational types of appeal." As Weaver puts it, those who use this source "are under a temptation to play too much upon the fears of their audience by stressing the awful nature of some consequence."[60]

Throughout Kass's writings, he appears to base his arguments on shared concepts—of personhood, nature, and so on. Yet when evaluating possible technological interventions, he shifts away from what Weaver thought the most natural appeal for a conservative, genus, and toward the source of consequences.[61] For Weaver, such arguments entail a prediction of "usually extremely desirable or undesirable results," which are presented as the "determining factor in deciding whether or not to adopt the proposed action."[62] This means that an argument that uses consequences can move either from cause to effect or effect to cause:

> The politician argues that, if he is elected (cause), there will be better government (effect); he argues that the present corruption in government (effect) must have been produced by a corrupt administration (cause); and that his happy home, successful career, and firm church and civic affiliations are clear signs that he will administer the office he seeks wisely and honestly.[63]

One finds the move from effect to cause in several famous examples in bioethics. In "Character, Virtue and Self-interest in the Ethics of the Professions," Edmund Pellegrino begins by characterizing the "moral malaise" in the learned professions today and argues that its cause is not external factors like "commercialization, competition, government regulation, malpractice, advertising, public and media hostility, and a host of other inimical socio-economic forces," but rather deficiencies in character and virtue.[64] As mentioned in the discussion of historical retrodiction, Ezekiel Emanuel argues that the irresolvable nature of moral dilemmas in modern medicine "can be traced to the liberal political philosophy that informs our society's laws, policies, and practices."[65] And Robert Zussman, in *Intensive Care: Medical Ethics and the Medical Profession*, argues that medical ethics is not a response to moral problems in contemporary medicine but is itself the effect of a decline in medical authority.[66]

Unlike these examples, Kass' arguments typically move in the opposite direction: from cause to effect. Consider how Kass argues in relation to the issues of prenatal diagnosis and genetic counseling. Kass begins his argument by claiming that the topic is difficult to address without also taking into account one's position on abortion. Kass makes a number of general statements that he thinks "nearly everyone" would agree with, including that, because abortion is a "moral issue," anyone who is either "seeking or refusing an abortion can expect to be asked" to provide some justification for that decision.[67] Based on what may strike some as a highly unusual statement on consensus concerning abortion, Kass concludes it follows that first, a fetus has a moral claim to be free from violence because it is "a living being" and, second, any act that would terminate the pregnancy must only be done so with some explicit justification.[68] He then focuses on the ethics of aborting a fetus because it is "defective." Kass then provides his argument against aborting defective fetuses in relation to what he terms the "Living Defective," that "those abnormals who escape the net of detection and abortion."[69] At this point, he moves from the indicative mood (cause) to the potential mood (likely effect). He laments how the parents of a living defective will treat this child, which he argues will be as a "second-class specimen," and remarks how the "abnormal child may also feel resentful."[70] This concern over how a new medical technology used in reproduction will affect the life of the children who are born through it is a common pattern in Kass's bioethical arguments: against the benefits of IVF, he lists an entire series of potential negative consequences, both scientific and social;[71] in his argument against reproductive cloning, one of his central claims is that the cloned individuals will have profound identity problems.[72]

This is not the only way to argue against cloning. In George Annas' argument against human cloning, for example, he draws primarily from the source of genus.

> Cloning is replication, not reproduction, and represents a different in kind not in degree in the manner in which human beings reproduce. Thus, although the constitutional right not to reproduce would seem to apply with equal force to a right not to replicate, to the extent that there is a constitutional right to reproduce (if one is able to), it seems unlikely that existing privacy or liberty doctrine would extend this right to replication by cloning.[73]

To be fair to Kass, one should note that there is, in his arguments, an interrelationship between consequences and the genus sources of argument: the consequences he believes we should be concerned with are those that entail a departure from what he considers to be "natural." To take a different example, we can see the way genus and consequences are entangled in Kass' criticism of enhancement technology when he states that,

> there is a sense that the "naturalness" of means matters. It lies not in the fact that the assisting drugs and devices are artifacts, but in the danger of violating or deforming the deep structure of natural human activity. In most of our ordinary efforts at self-improvement, either by practice or training or study, we sense the relation between our doings and the resulting improvement, between the means used and the end sought.[74]

Another example of an argument from consequences can be found in Dan Brock's analysis of what is often referred to as physician-assisted dying, but was called "voluntary active euthanasia" at the time of his essay. After distinguishing his focus from other forms of physician involvement in the death of patients, such as involuntary active euthanasia, physician-assisted suicide, and passive euthanasia (withdrawal of treatment), Brock summarizes the argument for voluntary active euthanasia based on individual self-determination and well-being—and then includes its opposing view, the notion that euthanasia is the "deliberate killing of an innocent person." The majority of Brock's essay, however, takes a public policy perspective on the issue. From this vantage, Brock is solely concerned with an evaluation based on consequences. He looks at the potential good consequences of allowing this action, the potential bad consequences of allowing it, and finally, whether it might lead to a "slippery slope" if it were legalized. Before providing a coda concerning whether physicians should have a role in this action if it were permitted, Brock summarizes his analysis:

> I have cited both good and bad consequences that have been thought likely from a policy change permitting voluntary active euthanasia and have tried to evaluate their likelihood and relative importance. Nevertheless, as I noted earlier, reasonable disagreement remains both about the consequences of permitting euthanasia and about which of these consequences are more important. The depth and strength of public and professional debate about whether, all things considered, permitting euthanasia would be desirable or undesirable reflects these disagreements. While my own view is that the balance of considerations supports permitting the practice, my principal purpose here has been to clarify the main issues.[75]

Weaver held a dim view of the argument from consequences. While he admitted that we all, at times, will need to make arguments based on this source, he saw it ultimately as the expression of the pragmatist. In his Platonic worldview, this appeal to a world "in flux" fell short of higher truths; it was an appeal to the "realm of becoming" rather than to the realm of being.[76]

RHETORICAL-HISTORICAL

Shortly before he died, Weaver identified another source of argument called rhetorical-historical. This argument entails an appeal to historical change in relation to some genus or definition, which becomes "a synthesis of principle with cause and circumstance."[77] While this may seem very much within the "realm of becoming," Weaver argues that this source does not indicate a "pragmatic argument with whatever fact comes last tipping the balance. History has extent and depth, revealing the lines of growth over a period of time."[78] A good example in bioethics of an argument made with this source is H. Tristram Engelhardt's *The Foundations of Bioethics*, which, as observed in the chapter on history and retrodiction, is based on the historical failure of the Enlightenment in Western philosophy. Engelhardt's argument is an admission that the philosophical project to find a secular, that is, based purely on reason, foundation for bioethics has been shown to have failed. As Engelhardt states in his preface: "I have endeavored to find grounds for establishing by reason a particular view of the good life and securing by general rational arguments the authority of its establishment. To my dismay and sorrow, such have not been available."[79] While Engelhardt wishes to establish the genus of a content-full, secular ethic, he is left only with a processual one, an ethic that offers little beyond grounds for agreement to permit new medical interventions. Yet *The Foundations of Bioethics* also has a "sibling" monograph, drawn upon less often in the discipline. *The Foundations of Christian Bioethics* represents Engelhardt's attempt to provide the content he could not provide in a secular philosophical framework:

> While addressing the sparse secular morality that can bind moral strangers when they are deaf to God, both editions [of *The Foundations of Bioethics*] stressed that there should be, and indeed that there truly is, the thick morality of moral friends. This volume speaks to what that morality should be.[80]

In this way Engelhardt maintains Weaver's hierarchy of value in terms of argumentative sources; above the changing principles of human history resides the more consistent authority of religious ideals. This new form of bioethics takes as its source of argument an appeal to the authority of Christian scripture, leaving behind the failure of the rhetorical-historical basis used in *The Foundations of Bioethics*.

CIRCUMSTANCES

The criteria established by the Ad Hoc Committee of the Harvard Medical School to Examine the Definition of Brain Death have been discussed earlier in relation to the rhetorical power of dissociation. The essay issued by that committee in 1968 begins: "Our primary purpose is to redefine irreversible coma as a new criterion for death."[81] From that opening, one might assume that the source of the committee's argument on brain death is one of definition, and will go on to define a shared genus. But the rest of the paragraph indicates that the committee is not so much providing a new ontological definition of death as providing the characteristics and legal issues surrounding the use of the brain's "health" as an indication of death.

> There are two reasons why there is need for a definition: (1) Improvements in resuscitative and supportive measures have led to increased efforts to save those who are desperately injured. Sometimes these efforts have only partial success so that the result is an individual whose heart continues to beat but

> whose brain is irreversibly damaged. The burden is great on patients who suffer permanent loss of intellect, on their families, on the hospitals, and on those in need of hospital beds already occupied by these comatose patients. (2) Obsolete criteria for the definition of death can lead to controversy in obtaining organs for transplantation.[82]

The justification for using the status of brain activity as the locus of determining death is based, thus, on the "burden" created by technological interventions that keep blood circulation and respiration going, and the "controversy" of obtaining organs for transplants from such individuals. As they further explain, "If the characteristics [of 'irreversible coma'] can be defined in satisfactory terms, translatable into action—and we believe this is possible—then several problems will either disappear or will become more readily soluble."[83] We see here that the argument made in this report is not based on an appeal to or creation of a genus, which would mean a justification based on claims about the essential nature of something. Instead, this is a pragmatic argument, one mounted in response to two technological changes: artificial respiration and organ transplantation. The authors are not arguing that we need to use the brain's status as the definition of death because our prior definition was illogical or somehow flawed, but that this prior definition causes difficulty in the current social and medical environment.

The Harvard committee's report is a good example of what Weaver refers to as justification through circumstances. Weaver characterizes this as an argument that "merely reads the circumstances—the 'facts standing around'—and accepts them as coercive, or allows them to dictate the decision."[84] Weaver considered it the lowest source, ethically speaking, for it was for him the "least philosophical" and, in its yielding to wayward context, "a surrender of reason."[85] Compared to one based on consequences, arguments from circumstances do not even attempt to predict the results of a particular action; they "only [make] an estimate of current conditions or pressures."[86] The distinction becomes clear when we compare the committee's definition to the one proposed by James Bernat, Charles Culver, and Bernard Gert, whose definition of brain death relies on an appeal to genus. "'Death' . . . is not a technical term," they write,

> but a common term in everyday use. We believe that a proper understanding of the ordinary meaning of the word or concept of death must be developed before a medical criterion of death is chosen. We must decide what is commonly meant by death before physicians can decide how to measure it.[87]

Another example of what could be classified as an argument based on circumstance is in Alison Jaggar's argument advocating the legalization of abortion. In "Abortion and a Woman's Right to Decide," Jaggar argues that because we live in a society in which women have been given the primary responsibility of caring for children and thus are the ones primarily affected by their birth, it should be up to women to decide whether to have children.

> The moral right to abortion for which I argue, however, is not a universal or absolute one enjoyed by all women, regardless of their social situation. Rather, it is a right whose existence depends on certain contingent features of the social situation in which women find themselves. Within our society, I shall argue, conditions are such that most women have a moral right to abortion, and, consequently, this right should be guaranteed by law. However, it is possible to describe other societies in which women do not have the sole moral right to decide on abortion, and indeed even within our own society there may be some women who do not have that right.[88]

Jaggar explicitly constructs her argument on what she acknowledges are contingent social conditions and even concedes that her argument would no longer be valid in a society in which men were the primary caretakers of children. Jaggar reinforces the essay's appeal to circumstances in her assessment of its strengths: namely, she does not need to entertain questions about the moral status of the fetus or the right to autonomy over one's body (the central concern of the "pro-life" and "pro-choice" positions, respectively). By steering clear of these poles, she sees her position as "acceptable to people of most shades of political opinion."[89]

In her later essay "Regendering the U.S. Abortion Debate," Jaggar reflects on her earlier argument in support of abortion, which she believes makes a "feminist" argument for abortion rights. She contrasts this approach with a "nonfeminist" argument,[90] taking Michael Tooley's renowned essay "Abortion and Infanticide" as her example. Whereas Jaggar's argument is based on the particular social conditions of our current world, Tooley's rests on defining a fetus as something other than a person, meaning that a fetus should not be considered to have "rights" in the manner that persons do.[91] Tooley's argument depends upon the notion of a stable genus of "persons" and his belief that a fetus does not exist in this category—regardless of circumstances. Comparing the argument concerning brain death from the Harvard committee to that of Bernat, Culver, and Gert, and the argument for abortion from Jaggar to that of Tooley, one can see how different making the "present circumstance the overbearing consideration"[92] in an argument is from an argument from genus.

SOURCE AND DESCRIPTION

The difference between how Jaggar and Tooley characterize the issue of abortion demonstrates how the same issue can be redescribed in relation to a different source, even when both parties prescribe the same course of action. Sources are thus not simply a method of justification but also a guide to how moral problems are understood. Jaggar's form of justification relies upon her description of abortion in relation to social expectations for women. Her article attends to the social circumstances of our society after a child is born. For Jaggar, one need not spend any time characterizing the fetus in terms of its ontology; the overriding consideration is the burden the existence of the child will have on its mother. "Every woman's life is enormously affected by the birth of her child," yet "the effect of a new births on the rest our society is small."[93] Tooley's essay, on the other hand, examines in detail the categories of rights and selfhood, without a concern in the description of any particular society in which this happens. Weaver recognized that the source selected for an argument is entangled with a distinct description of the world. In "Language is Sermonic" Weaver asserts that being aware of the chosen source enables us to see that the reader is not asked "to follow a valid reasoning form but to respond to some presentation of reality."[94]

NOTES

1. Lisa Sowle Cahill, "Abortion and Argument by Analogy," *Horizons* 9, no. 2 (1982); B. Hofmann, J. H. Solbakk, and S. Holm, "Teaching Old Dogs New Tricks: The Role of Analogies in Bioethical Analysis and Argumentation Concerning New Technologies," *Theoretical Medicine and Bioethics* 27, no. 5 (2006); Robert Hunt Sprinkle, "Bioethics Without Analogy," in *Clinical Ethics and the Necessity of Stories: Essays in Honor of Richard M. Zaner*, ed. Osborne P. Wiggins and Annette C. Allen (Dordrecht: Springer, 2010), 71–85.
2. Albert R. Jonsen and Stephen Edelston Toulmin, *The Abuse of Casuistry: A History of Moral Reasoning* (Berkeley, CA: University of California Press, 1988), 297.
3. James F. Childress, *Practical Reasoning in Bioethics*, Medical Ethics Series (Bloomington, IN: Indiana University Press, 1997), 18.
4. Cahill, "Abortion and Argument by Analogy," 278.
5. Peter Singer, *Animal Liberation: The Definitive Classic of the Animal Movement*, Updated ed. (New York: Ecco, 2009), 6.
6. Richard M. Weaver, *The Ethics of Rhetoric* (Battleboro, VT: Echo Point Books & Media, 2011), 222.
7. Roger Gilles, "Richard Weaver Revisited: Rhetoric Left, Right, and Middle," *Rhetoric Review* 15, no. 1 (1996): 130.
8. Weaver, *The Ethics of Rhetoric,* 55.
9. Weaver, *The Ethics of Rhetoric,* 58.
10. Sonja K. Foss, "Abandonment of Genus: The Evolution of Political Rhetoric," *Communication Studies* 33, no. 2 (1982) 370.
11. Weaver, *The Ethics of Rhetoric,* 57.

12. Kevin Wm Wildes, "The Priesthood of Bioethics and the Return of Casuistry," *Journal of Medicine and Philosophy* 18, no. 1 (1993): 33–49.

13. It should be noted that Weaver's typology of sources, or what he sometimes referred to as "topics" vary in relation to the time period in which Weaver was writing. For example, in his book on composition, Weaver argued that there were eight sources: Richard M. Weaver, *Composition: A Course in Writing and Rhetoric* (New York: Holt, 1957), 123–135 and in his essay "Language is Sermonic" he lists only four: Richard M. Weaver, *Language is Sermonic: Richard M. Weaver on the Nature of Rhetoric*, ed. Richard L. Johannesen, Rennard Strickland, and Ralph T. Eubanks (Baton Rouge, LA: Louisiana State University Press, 1985), 209.

14. Weaver, *Language is Sermonic: Richard M. Weaver on the Nature of Rhetoric,* 214.

15. Weaver, *The Ethics of Rhetoric,* 83.

16. John R. E. Bliese, "Richard Weaver's Axiology of Argument," *Southern Speech Communication Journal* 44, no. 3 (1979): 275–288.

17. Sonja K. Foss, Karen A. Foss, and Robert Trapp, *Contemporary Perspectives on Rhetoric*, 3rd ed. (Prospect Heights, IL: Waveland Press, 2002), 166.

18. Weaver, *Composition: A Course in Writing and Rhetoric,* 132.

19. Weaver, *Composition: A Course in Writing and Rhetoric,* 133.

20. Weaver, *Composition: A Course in Writing and Rhetoric,* 133.

21. Allen Verhey, *Reading the Bible in the Strange World of Medicine* (Grand Rapids, MI: W.B. Eerdmans Pub. Co., 2003), 74.

22. Verhey, *Reading the Bible in the Strange World of Medicine,* 76.

23. Verhey, *Reading the Bible in the Strange World of Medicine,* 33.

24. Eloise Rosenblatt, "Book Review—Reading the Bible in the Strange World of Medicine," *Health Progress* (July–August 2005): 67.

25. Weaver, *Language Is Sermonic: Richard M. Weaver on the Nature of Rhetoric,* 210.

26. Leon R. Kass, "Practicing Ethics: Where's the Action?," *The Hastings Center Report* 20, no. 1 (1990): 7. Cf. Renée C. Fox, Judith P. Swazey, and Judith C. Watkins, *Observing Bioethics* (Oxford: Oxford University Press, 2008), 37–38.

27. Weaver, *Composition: A Course in Writing and Rhetoric,* 133.

28. See Weaver, *Composition: A Course in Writing and Rhetoric,* 132–133.

29. Arthur W. Frank, *The Wounded Storyteller: Body, Illness, and Ethics* (Chicago, IL: University of Chicago Press, 1995), 137.

30. Frank, *The Wounded Storyteller: Body, Illness, and Ethics*, 137.

31. John D. Arras, "Nice Story, But So What? Narrative and Justification in Ethics," in *Stories and Their Limits: Narrative Approaches to Bioethics*, ed. Hilde Lindemann Nelson (New York: Routledge, 2014), 82.

32. Howard Brody, *Stories of Sickness*, 2nd ed. (Oxford: Oxford University Press, 2003), 156.

33. Thomas Tomlinson, *Methods in Medical Ethics: Critical Perspectives* (Oxford: Oxford University Press, 2012), 129–130.

34. Brody, *Stories of Sickness,* 160 note 5.

35. Tomlinson, *Methods in Medical Ethics: Critical Perspectives,* 146.

36. Tom Regan, *The Case for Animal Rights*, Updated with a new pref. ed. (Berkeley, CA: University of California Press, 2004).

37. Carl Cohen, "In Defense of the Use of Animals," in *The Animal Rights Debate*, ed. Carl Cohen and Tom Regan (Lanham, MD: Rowman & Littlefield, 2006), 22–23.

38. Weaver, *The Ethics of Rhetoric,* 56.

39. Weaver, *The Ethics of Rhetoric,* 86.

40. Cohen, "In Defense of the Use of Animals," 17.

41. Cohen, "In Defense of the Use of Animals," 19, note 1.

42. Cohen, "In Defense of the Use of Animals," 30.

43. Weaver, *The Ethics of Rhetoric,* 56.

44. Weaver, *Composition: A Course in Writing and Rhetoric,* 126.

45. Weaver, *The Ethics of Rhetoric,* 86.

46. David Zarefsky, "Presidential Rhetoric and the Power of Definition," *Presidential Studies Quarterly* 34, no. 3 (2004): 612.

47. Leon Kass, *Toward a More Natural Science: Biology and Human Affairs* (New York: Free Press, 1985), xii.

48. Gregory E. Kaebnick, *Humans in Nature: The World as We Find It and the World as We Create It* (Oxford: Oxford University Press, 2014).

49. Lawrence J. Schneiderman and Nancy Jecker, *Wrong Medicine: Doctors, Patients, and Futile Treatment* (Baltimore, MD: Johns Hopkins University Press, 1995), 8.

50. Schneiderman and Jecker, *Wrong Medicine: Doctors, Patients, and Futile Treatment,* 11.

51. Thaddeus Mason Pope, "Review of Lawrence J. Schneiderman and Nancy S. Jecker, Wrong Medicine: Doctors, Patients, and Futile Treatment," *American Journal of Bioethics* 12, no. 1 (2012): 50.

52. Richard L. Johannesen, "Richard M. Weaver on Standards for Ethical Rhetoric," *Communication Studies* 29, no. 2 (1978): 127–137.

53. Schneiderman and Jecker, *Wrong Medicine: Doctors, Patients, and Futile Treatment,* 8.

54. Schneiderman and Jecker, *Wrong Medicine: Doctors, Patients, and Futile Treatment,* 11.

55. Schneiderman and Jecker, *Wrong Medicine: Doctors, Patients, and Futile Treatment,* 17.

56. Margrit Shildrick, *Leaky Bodies and Boundaries: Feminism, Postmodernism and (Bio)ethics* (London: Routledge, 1997).

57. Richard Twine, "Constructing Critical Bioethics by Deconstructing Culture/nature Dualism," *Medicine, Health Care and Philosophy* 8 (2005).

58. Gregory E. Pence, *Who's Afraid of Human Cloning?* (Lanham, MD: Rowman & Littlefield, 1998), 27.

59. It should be noted that some see a difference in Weaver's typology between "consequences" and "cause and effect" as sources. Richard Johannesen, in his summary of the typology, refers to consequences as separate from cause and effect. He sees argument from consequences as "a subvariant of causal reasoning." Richard L. Johannesen, "Richard Weaver's View of Rhetoric and Criticism," *Southern Journal*

of Communication 32, no. 2 (1966): 133–145. One finds in other summaries of Weaver's typology of sources that the two are used interchangeably.

60. Weaver, *Language is Sermonic: Richard M. Weaver on the Nature of Rhetoric,* 214.

61. One can see this interplay of movement from genus to consequences in Kass's most well-known work, *Toward a More Natural Science: Biology and Human Affairs*. Kass, *Toward a More Natural Science: Biology and Human Affairs.*

62. Johannesen, "Richard Weaver's View of Rhetoric and Criticism," 142.

63. Manuel Bilsky et al., "Looking for an Argument," *College English* (1953): 214.

64. Edmund D. Pellegrino, "Character, Virtue and Self-Interest in the Ethics of the Professions," *The Journal of Contemporary Health Law & Policy* 5 (1989): 53.

65. Ezekiel J. Emanuel, *The Ends of Human Life: Medical Ethics in a Liberal Polity* (Cambridge, MA: Harvard University Press, 1991), 7.

66. Robert Zussman, *Intensive Care: Medical Ethics and the Medical Profession* (Chicago, IL: University of Chicago Press, 1994).

67. Leon R. Kass, "Implications of Prenatal Diagnosis for the Human Right to Life," in *Biomedical Ethics and the Law*, ed. James M. Humber and Robert F. Almeder (Boston, MA: Springer, 1979), 336.

68. Kass, "Implications of Prenatal Diagnosis for the Human Right to Life," 336–337.

69. Kass, "Implications of Prenatal Diagnosis for the Human Right to Life," 339.

70. Kass, "Implications of Prenatal Diagnosis for the Human Right to Life," 340.

71. Leon R. Kass, "Making Babies—the New Biology and the Old Morality," *The Public Interest* 26 (1972): 18.

72. Leon R. Kass, "The Wisdom of Repugnance: Why We Should Ban the Cloning of Humans," *New Republic* 216, no. 22 (1997): 22.

73. George J. Annas, "Scientific Discoveries and Cloning: Challenges for Public Policy," in *Flesh of my flesh: The Ethics of Cloning Humans*, ed. Gregory E. Pence (Lanham, MD: Rowman & Littlefield, 1998), 80.

74. Leon R. Kass, "Ageless Bodies, Happy Souls: Biotechnology and the Pursuit of Perfection," *The New Atlantis* 1 (2003): 22.

75. Dan W. Brock, "Active Voluntary Euthanasia," *Hastings Center Report* 22, no. 2 (March–April 1992): 21.

76. Johannesen, "Richard Weaver's View of Rhetoric and Criticism," 142.

77. Bliese, "Richard Weaver's Axiology of Argument," 280.

78. Richard M. Weaver, "Two Orators," *Modern Age* 14, no. 3 (1970): 232.

79. H. Tristram Engelhardt, *The Foundations of Bioethics*, 2nd ed. (New York: Oxford University Press, 1996), viii.

80. H. Tristram Engelhardt, *The Foundations of Christian Bioethics* (Lisse: Swets & Zeitlinger, 2000), xvi.

81. Henry K. Beecher, "A Definition of Irreversible Coma: Report of the Ad Hoc Committee of the Harvard Medical School to Examine the Definition of Brain Death," *Journal of the American Medical Association* 205, no. 6 (1968): 85.

82. Beecher, "A Definition of Irreversible Coma: Report of the Ad Hoc Committee of the Harvard Medical School to Examine the Definition of Brain Death," 85.

83. Beecher, "A Definition of Irreversible Coma: Report of the Ad Hoc Committee of the Harvard Medical School to Examine the Definition of Brain Death," 85.

84. Weaver, *The Ethics of Rhetoric,* 57.

85. Weaver, *Language Is Sermonic: Richard M. Weaver on the Nature of Rhetoric,* 57.

86. Weaver, *The Ethics of Rhetoric,* 57.

87. James L. Bernat, Charles M. Culver, and Bernard Gert, "On the Definition and Criterion of Death," *Annals of Internal Medicine* 94, no. 3 (1981): 389.

88. Alison M. Jaggar, "Abortion and a Woman's Right to Decide," in *Living With Contradictions, ed. Alison M. Jaggar* (Boulder, CO: Westview Press, 1994), 281.

89. Jaggar, "Abortion and a Woman's Right to Decide," 281.

90. Alison M. Jaggar, "Regendering the US Abortion Debate," *Journal of Social Philosophy* 28, no. 1 (1997): 127–140.

91. Michael Tooley, "Abortion and Infanticide," *Philosophy & Public Affairs* (1972): 37–65.

92. Weaver, *The Ethics of Rhetoric,* 57.

93. Jaggar, "Abortion and a Woman's Right to Decide," 284.

94. Weaver, *Language Is Sermonic: Richard M. Weaver on the Nature of Rhetoric,* 210.

Chapter 7

Hypertextuality

In the discussion of anagnorisis, one of my examples was Robert Veatch's redescription of the Hippocratic tradition in *A Theory of Medical Ethics*. It has been argued that this 1981 work was the first attempt to provide a "full exposition of the theoretical underpinnings" of the new field of bioethics.[1] Whether that claim is true or not, it is a prime example of a key genre within bioethics writing, which I will refer to as "foundational texts." Foundational texts are those works in bioethics that have as their central aim the establishment of a theoretical base for the resolution of moral problems within biomedicine—and which accomplish that aim through an appeal to a prior foundational moral system. This category includes a wide variety of theoretical positions, many of which have already been discussed: the contractualism of Veatch's book, the casuistry of Al Jonsen and Stephen Toulmin's *The Abuse of Casuistry*, the principlism of Tom Beauchamp and James Childress' *Principles of Biomedical Ethics*, the communitarianism of Ezekiel Emanuel's *The Ends of Human Life*, the virtue ethics of David Thomasma and Edmund Pellegrino's *The Virtues in Medical Practice*, the phenomenology of Richard Zaner's *Ethics and the Clinical Encounter*, and the postmodern ethics of Arthur Frank's *The Wounded Storyteller*. When of monograph length, as texts in this genre tend to be, the works propose a global solution to all moral problems that arise in medical practice, or in some cases provide an explanation for why there is no global solution, as in Tristram Engelhardt's minimalist secular ethic in *The Foundation of Bioethics*.

Although *A Theory of Medical Ethics* may be the field's first foundational text, Veatch's opening paragraph acknowledges that it must be appreciated within a plethora of other works—including "[s]cores of volumes, hundreds of journal articles, and thousands of courses."[2] By placing his text in conversation with other texts, Veatch is making explicit the manner in which his work (as all texts) needs to be understood in terms of its relation to these other texts, which surround, precede, and pervade his argument for a general theory of bioethics. *A Theory of Medical Ethics* engages in a form of dialogue not only with the Hippocratic oath, but also with such texts as Paul Ramsey's *The Patient as Person*, Thomas Percival's code of ethics, letters in medical journals, Immanuel Kant's *Groundwork of the Metaphysic of Morals*, the Talmud, American legal cases, John Stuart Mill's *On Liberty*, the United Nations' Declaration of Human Rights, ethics case narrations, the Zoroastrian *Avesta*, and Aristotle's *Nichomachean Ethics*. Bioethics arguments, like all texts, are an assortment of preceding texts; this interweaving is known by literary critics as "intertextuality." And while the sources named above are explicitly cited by Veatch as informing his ethic of medicine, literary critics are quick to point out that the concept of intertextuality does not end with explicit citation or even with the discernible influences of a particular text. First coined by Julia Kristeva, intertextuality as we have come to understand it entails the way that *all* texts are constructed out of the fragments of prior texts—how they are all, to quote Roland Barthes, "quotations without inverted commas."[3]

Literary critic Gérard Genette defined it more narrowly, however. In this chapter I follow Genette in placing intertextuality underneath the umbrella term of *transtextuality*, or "all that sets the text in a relationship, whether obvious or concealed, with other texts."[4] Genette identifies five types of transtextual relationships: architextuality, intertextuality, paratextuality, metatextuality, and hypertextuality. Architextuality involves a text's relationship to prior texts in terms of such features as "types of discourse, modes of enunciation, literary genres";[5] the bioethics texts cited above can be grouped together because they share the same architextuality, that is, as examples of the foundational genre in bioethics. Intertextuality, as Genette uses it,[6] refers to a relationship that involves the "copresence" of two or more texts, most often through direct quotation. This form of transtextuality can be noted in forms other than literature, as when George Crumb in his musical work *Black Angels* "quotes" a part of Franz Schubert's *Death and the Maiden*. In written work, however, quotation marks are necessary. Without them, the status of the relationship between the two remains one of intertextuality, but the silent quotation of the prior text, if discovered, would be considered a form of plagiarism. Paratextuality refers to those texts that are peripheral to a text, such as titles, epigraphs, and external reviews, and they often function to condition a particular response to a text. The subtitle of a book as a "medical thriller" acts as a threshold text for the reader that, in turn, creates expectations for how the text should be experienced. When the directors of the 1996 film *Fargo* began the film with a screen title "based on a true story," which it was not, they influenced how the audience, who had no way of detecting this deception, responded to the film's plot. Metatextuality is Genette's term for what is most often referred to as the commentary of one text on another. As Genette notes, this type of relationship can exist even if the other text is rarely if ever explicitly mentioned; for example, "Hegel, in *The Phenomenology of the Mind*, allusively and almost silently evoke[s] Denis Diderot's *Neveu de Rameau*," although Hegel does in the work have two instances of intertextual direct quotations from the work.[7] Hypertextuality, the fifth form of transtextuality, is a text that has been in some manner "grafted" onto another text. The classic examples that Genette provides are the relationship of Homer's *Odyssey* to Virgil's *Aeneid* and James Joyce's *Ulysses*. Though each text is highly distinctive, both texts, which Genette refers to as the hypertexts, have a direct relationship to Homer's work, the hypotext. They are not commentaries on Homer but are still in some way derived from him.

Bioethics authors use these last two types of transtextuality to clear a space for their arguments. There is nothing unique about this combination, as it forms the central transtextual relationship in academic discourse: authors comment metatextually on a hypertext that they themselves have constructed through redescription. The bioethicist creates the text, which is a hypertextual transformation of a prior text, which is then criticized through their commentary. This formula is especially important for those attempting to argue for a novel philosophical foundation for the discipline. In Veatch's book, the entire first part is a metatextual—and critical—examination of the Hippocratic tradition, the Judeo-Christian tradition, and the modern western secular tradition. In this structure, Veatch's text expresses one of the conventions of the foundational genre; he frames his theoretical position in opposition to other moral traditions. A conviction running through most foundational texts is the sense that we are still facing moral problems, so the present theoretical structure has not provided enough guidance. Foundational texts, including Veatch's, stage a struggle between this earlier theoretical position and their own—an epic contest between two moral perspectives. Through metatextuality, Jonsen and Toulmin in *The Abuse of Casuistry* create an agonistic struggle between top-down principles and a bottom-up, case-based approach. In *No Longer Patient*, Sherwin comments on what she refers to as the "mainstream moral theory" of Kant and utilitarianism before offering her feminist "contextual ethics" as a better alternative. These commentaries, however, enact a metatextual relationship with an argument of the bioethicist's *own* construction.

This chapter will look at the way these two forms of hypertextuality permit the bioethicist to describe the hypotext as inadequate, establishing the need for the hypertextual replacement by the author and laying the groundwork for the rhetorical form that the replacement will take.

CONTINUATION IN BIOETHICS

In *Palimpsests*, Genette uses Virgil's *Aeneid* and Joyce's *Ulysses* to help explicate the various and complex ways a hypertext can transform the hypotext. As Genette explains, "Joyce extracts from it [Homer's *Odyssey*] a pattern of actions and relationships, which he treats altogether in a different style. Virgil appropriates a certain style, which he applies to a different action."[8] Or take, for example, two twentieth-century film adaptations of Jane Austen's novel 1815 *Emma*: Amy Heckerling's *Clueless* (1995) and Douglas McGrath's *Emma* (1996). McGrath's transformation is primarily located in the medium of presentation; other than shifting from print to film, he strives to provide an accurate re-presentation of the plot, characters, and time period of Austen's novel. Heckerling's film maintains the key characters and plot for the most part, but sets the story in a contemporary Beverly Hills high school. *Clueless* thus transforms *Emma* through the medium, the time period, and the setting, yet still attempts to maintain the story's themes, tone, and meaning. Film is a particularly good example of transformation because of its temporal constraints, which limit the elements of the story that can be related. While filmic transformations tend to entail reduction, other media can accommodate expansions, as in the elaboration of biblical stories in novels such as José Saramago's *Cain* and Thomas Mann's *Joseph and His Brothers*. Bioethics texts also involve elements of reduction and expansion of prior texts.

Let us start with their use of expansion, and specifically the expansion of a prior moral theory into the field of bioethics. This practice is best captured by Genette's classification of one type of expansion he refers to as "continuation," by which the hypotext is augmented by additional text in the hypertext. Genette's discussion of this form of augmentation starts with hypertexts that are constructed to complete a hypotext that was never finished. For example, Charles Dickens' serialized novel *The Mystery of Edwin Drood* was left unfinished because the author died before completing it, but subsequent authors have supplied their own conclusions to the work. Genette observes, however, that continuations have been produced even when the author *did* bring the original work to completion: "[o]ne can always decide that a work which is finished and published as such by its author is nevertheless in need of a prolongation or a completion."[9] Virgil's *Aeneid* is, for Genette, an example of a continuation that attempts to fill in gaps in the narrative of the *Iliad*.[10] The canon of Sherlock Holmes mysteries is another major launching point for continuations. Arthur Conan Doyle himself created a continuation of the story of Sherlock Holmes when, after killing off his protagonist in "The Final Problem," he responded to popular demand—first by writing a Holmes story that took place prior to the events of his death, and then by writing the story "The Adventure of the Empty House," in which Holmes' death is actually revealed to have been false. Since Doyle's death, stories concerning his detective have expanded well beyond the original canon, including stories focusing on a retired Holmes like Laurie King's *The Beekeeper's Apprentice* and Mitch Cullin's *A Slight Trick of the Mind*. Other continuations of literary classics include the radical reframing of *Hamlet* by Tom Stoppard in *Rosencrantz & Guildenstern Are Dead*, and Jean Rhys telling the backstory of *Jane Eyre*'s Mrs. Rochester in her novel *Wide Sargasso Sea*. Madeline Miller's *The Song of Achilles* elaborates the story of Achilles' relationship with Patroclus. These continuations illustrate the various forms of expansion identified by Genette: *proleptic* continuation, which provides a hypertext account of things that happen chronologically after the hypotext (as in the examples above of a retired Sherlock Holmes); *analeptic* continuation of things that happened before the hypotext (such as Rhys' story about the young woman who would become Mrs. Rochester); *elliptic* continuation, which fills in gaps in the narrative (as in Miller's focus on Patroclus); and *paraleptic* continuations that provide lateral explications of things that occur in the hypotext (as in Stoppard's play, which exists alongside *Hamlet*).[11]

Continuation is so important to bioethics because the discipline tends not to develop novel moral theories as much as it takes prior theories and extends them into the moral issues of medical practice. In this way, bioethics texts can be thought of as philosophical continuations—additions to the plot of philosophical ideas of a prior thinker. Veatch's book is a transformation of the social contract theory of John Locke and Thomas Hobbes. Joseph Fins, Matthew Bacchetta, and Franklin Miller's concept of "clinical pragmatism" is a transformation of the concept of inquiry developed by John Dewey. Laurie Zoloth's *Health Care and the Ethics of Encounter* transports Emmanuel Levinas' understanding of our obligations to the Other into the realm of healthcare rationing. And Zaner transforms the phenomenology of Edmund Husserl into a concern with the moral ground of clinical encounters. Each of these is an instance of the bioethicist taking a prior moral theory and extending it into a subject it had not addressed. For many, this extension is into a realm that the prior author had not imagined; it is difficult to believe that Dewey in his pragmatism in some manner forgot to include discussions of medical ethics. As Genette notes,

> The function of continuation, however, is not always to complete a work that has been left manifestly and, as it were, officially unfinished. One can always decide that a work which is finished and published as such by its author is nevertheless in need of a prolongation or a completion.[12]

Unlike Zaner's extension of phenomenology into clinical ethics, there are examples in bioethics in which part of the argument is that the prior hypertext was in fact incomplete (or inadequate). For example, Norman Daniels' monograph *Just Health Care* is in many ways a continuation of John Rawls' theory of justice into the realm of health care. As Daniels notes, however, Rawls' theory applies to

> individuals who are "normal, active, and fully cooperating members of society over the course of a complete life." . . . Such idealization allows Rawls to construct a theory of justice of the simpler, idealized case, and then to worry about extensions of the theory to contexts in which conditions are more realistic and people are not all normal. In effect, *there is no distributive theory for health care because no one is sick!*[13]

Daniels positions his particular transformation of Rawls as a necessary elaboration, filling in the gaps of logic and application that the original work left unaddressed. Similarly, Drew Leder in *The Distressed Body* provides a continuation of the hermeneutic method of Hans Gadamer, who had written on the hermeneutics of medicine but not on issues of bioethics. Leder refers to his continuation as "phenomenologically informed hermeneutics," an approach to bioethics that attends to "the embodied, contextualized situation of participants and practices" in contrast to the tendency in bioethics to start from abstract theory.[14] In *The Loyal Physician*, Griffin Trotter draws upon Josiah Royce's philosophy of loyalty as a foundation for the ethics of the medical profession. Directly citing Royce's claim in *The Philosophy of Loyalty* that "his theory provides a template for professional ethics" in general, Trotter explicitly acknowledges that his is a continuation of Royce's moral theory, and suggests that his work answers an invitation made by Royce.[15]

While these are all examples of a hypertextual amplification of a hypotext, there is another form of transformation at play here: the later authors must explicitly summarize, and thus necessarily reduce, the prior text. In *The Loyal Physician*, Griffin includes two chapters summarizing Royce's philosophy and, in particular, his concept of loyalty—conveyed, of course, through his own metatextual commentary; the rest of his book is devoted to extending Royce's loyalty into medical ethics. In relation to Royce's hypotext, then, Griffin begins with a reduction and finishes with an augmentation.

Less straightforwardly, continuations can at times result in a transformation that alters the original meaning of the hypotext. In *Bioethics as Practice*, Judith Andre notes how surprised she was to find that the idea of *autonomy*—which she had learned in her training as a philosopher—was translated in bioethics into a very different concept. Andre relates how, when autonomy was discussed prior to her entrance into the field of bioethics, it always meant

> the corresponding responsibility, and finally the right of human beings to choose the principles according to which they live. . . . Autonomy is not a matter of having a choice; it is an inner stance toward whatever choices one has.[16]

In the field of bioethics, however, Andre found a very different definition of the term. As Andre observes, those who are not trained as philosophers "understandably assume that 'autonomy' as it is used in bioethics is a direct, unaltered borrowing from the language of philosophers. Most philosophers know it is not, but cannot say exactly what it is."[17] Added to reductions of a theory that will then be augmented, Andre's example introduces a form of reduction that makes the prior text deficient or lacking, rather than just restricted to a specific arena. It is in this way that bioethicists (and most academics) claim the power to describe, or rather redescribe, a prior work with the aim of correcting it. In what follows, we will see how the redescription of prior works via reduction enables bioethicists to create the opponent they wish to engage.

THE INFIDELITY OF THE SUMMARY

Expansion, continuation, reduction: so far we have been looking at the way bioethicists' texts interact with prior texts from outside the world of biomedicine. Yet, as in all academic disciplines, bioethicists must also respond to—expand, continue, reduce—texts by other bioethicists. In *Health Care and the Ethics of Encounter*, Zoloth argues that the Jewish perspective on ethics she is advocating "offers resources" that "the feminist, Christian, and secular traditions have called for"—but have not so far been able to provide.[18] Leder argues that his "phenomenologically informed hermeneutics" is better able to respond to moral problems in the clinical setting because, unlike traditional bioethics' allegiance to abstractions, it attends closely to "real-life situations."[19] New theories or solutions must, in some manner, demonstrate that there is a problem with current methods of problem-solving.

Reduction is extremely helpful in this regard. In his discussion of reduction, Genette divides the concept into two forms: digest and summary. While both are reductions of the hypotext, a summary is also metatextual in that it provides a commentary upon the hypotext.[20] Tom Tomlinson's *Methods in Medical Ethics*—subtitled "Critical Perspectives"—is a work of summary and not digest, for Tomlinson is not merely explicating bioethics theories like care ethics, virtue ethics, and casuistry; he is grouping them together as methods that, while adding new qualities of moral analysis, nonetheless rely on abstract principles.[21] Most bioethics texts provide a summary of a prior hypotext, but it would be a mistake to think that the summary is independent of commentary, for the metatextual and hypertextual elements in bioethics texts are often entangled with each other. Like the historical frames discussed in chapter 1, there is an element of retrodiction in reduction-by-summary, in that the commentary to follow will, in some manner, reveal the shortcomings of the prior position.

In his analysis of literary adaptation, Robert Stam introduces the concept of "fidelity," noting that it is not uncommon for critics to evaluate a film adaptation in terms of whether it accurately expresses the text upon which it is based.[22] Stam, however, criticizes this impulse—and indeed the very notion of an adaptation being "unfaithful" to its source. Are we to believe that a novel contains some specific, nameable essence that cannot be left out? Furthermore, the medium of film and the medium of the novel are qualitatively different in their forms of communication, not to mention the limitations our culture has placed on their expression. (While there are exceptions like the Swedish experimental film *Logistics*, which runs to 51,420 minutes, most films come in under three hours, four at the most; novels do not share this particular limitation.) As opposed to fidelity, Stam favors Genette's notion of transformation as a more appropriate model for assessing film adaptations.

This preference becomes problematic in terms of academic texts, however. In academia, the notion of fidelity is essential because of the existence of subsequent metatextuality. Since the metatext waits for the text upon which it comments, and in bioethics, the text for which it is found wanting, the manner in which a hypertextual reduction is faithful to its hypotext becomes part of the argument in the work itself. Reductions become powerful sources of rhetorical persuasion primarily because they construct the very text upon which they then respond and invariably find wanting in some manner. This relationship of the metatext to the hypertext is similar to the relationship of the metatextual response to the bioethics case.[23] Take for example Veatch's key oppositional hypotext for *A Theory of Medical Ethics*, the Hippocratic Corpus. Veatch provides a colorful summary of the Hippocratic writings as akin to those of an insular cultish community. Tom Koch, in "The Hippocratic Thorn in Bioethics' Hide: Cults, Sects, and Strangeness," argues that Veatch incorrectly summarizes the corpus by portraying it in this manner. Rather than "bizarre, cultish, or even particularly dated," the Hippocratic texts, which Koch reminds us have been adopted widely outside their original context, signify an "ongoing" commitment to "patient care and health as a physician's primary duty."[24] Essentially, Koch is arguing that Veatch's summary is unfaithful to the original. Ascribing motivation for infidelity to the hypotext is unnecessary. Whether done purposely to misguide the reader or done inadvertently, without malice, the result is the same. The redescription leads the reader to see the hypotext as deficient in some fundamental manner, preparing the ground for a better theory or new moral position.

Somewhat complicating the idea of summaries, faithful or not, is the existence in bioethics of what Genette refers to as "pseudo-summaries." As Genette explains, a pseudo-summary is the "simulated summary of an imaginary text."[25] His chief example is Jorge Luis Borges' fictions, which contain summaries of works presented as real, but which in truth are texts that Borges himself has imagined. Bioethicists do not pass off imagined texts as real, of course, but they do at times construct an entity to be analyzed that may not exist, strictly speaking, in textual form. For instance, Margaret Walker in *Moral Understandings: A Feminist Study in Ethics* summarizes a model for moral theorizing that she refers to as the theoretical-juridical model, which she positions as a type of theoretical intertext for utilitarian, contractarian, Kantian, and rights-based approaches to moral theories.[26] And Edmund Pincoffs creates an entity he refers to as "quandary ethics," which he goes on to counter with his own virtue-based ethics.[27] These textual fictions for metatextual relations may become themselves the primary text for additional metatextual relations by other ethicists. So, we find Leigh Turner referring to Pincoffs' quandary ethics in his critique of the inattention to the ethos of *place* in medical facilities[28] and Hilde Lindemann and Howard Brody drawing upon Walker's "judicial-theoretical" model in their discussions of narrative ethics.[29]

Reductions, thus, can be, and perhaps always are, creative acts; they are not simply naïve summaries of prior arguments but creative representations that provide a space for new arguments. To further examine the importance that reduction has in bioethics, I will look at various digests of perhaps the most cited text in the field: Tom Beauchamp and James Childress' *Principles of Biomedical Ethics*. Richard Davis begins his essay "The Principlism Debate: A Critical Overview" by noting that principlism has become "[w]idely regarded as the most popular and influential product in the current bioethics marketplace," then asserts that the best example of this approach is Beauchamp and Childress' text.[30] The abiding dominance of the *Principles* in American bioethics is scrutinized by John Evans in "A Sociological Account of the Growth of Principlism."[31] Evans claims that principlism's rise owes to its utility for public policy: principlism's pragmatic structure had "the lure of calculability and predictability," which could be "replicated" across a large number of training and federal policies. Evans' argument is not in any manner a philosophical critique of the theory's strengths or weaknesses, but rather an attempt to explain through social theory how principlism rose to dominance within the world of bioethics in the United States. Regardless of how principlism came to dominate bioethics, a focus on principlism allows us to see how those advocating for a new theoretical position must in some manner demonstrate that principlism is, at the very least, inadequate in some manner or, at the most, hazardously erroneous as a framework for resolving moral biomedical problems. We should point out that it is in some ways incorrect to refer to *Principles of Biomedical Ethics* as a single text, for the authors published several editions, each with substantial revisions that expanded or revised elements of prior versions. Because of this, Beauchamp and Childress' text has become a bit of a moving target, its positions constantly shifting in response to critiques. This has led to a number of pseudo-summaries that were not always pseudo, as when critics attacked earlier versions of the now-revised theory. Critics have now had to identify which version of the text they are attacking, for subsequent editions may differ in ways that make their points less sharp. Furthermore, as John Arras has humorously noted, the text has come to resemble the aliens of *Star Trek*, who do not so much conquer people as assimilate them. When a critic submits

> a seemingly crippling broadside against the juggernaut of *PBE* from a casuist, narrativist, feminist, or pragmatist perspective, then than critique is promptly welcomed with open arms, trimmed of its excesses, and incorporated into the ever-expanding synthesis of the next edition.[32]

SUMMARIZING BEAUCHAMP AND CHILDRESS

As already discussed in the prior chapter on metaphor, Gert, Culver, and Clouser have been highly critical of Beauchamp and Childress' text. Their concept of a "common morality approach"[33] to bioethics has been developed over a number of their own texts, which themselves may be understood as a series of transformations. In 1982, Culver and Gert published a text titled *Philosophy in Medicine*, which took as one of its primary tasks improving the reader's understanding of concepts in medicine and psychiatry.[34] The medical world is filled with under-analyzed language and thus very much needs, according to Culver and Gert, to draw upon the methods of philosophy to address the gap. Few, I suspect, would consider Culver and Gert's book an example of the foundational genre within bioethics. The text does not provide a particular set of foundational concepts, rules, or methods by which the entire discipline should be directed. In 1997, Gert and Culver, now with K. Danner Clouser, published a radical rewriting of that 1982 text; the new one was titled *Bioethics: A Return to Fundamentals*. While much of the close analysis of concepts remained the same as when it appeared in *Philosophy in Medicine*, this new text provided a foundational approach to all of bioethics, essentially putting forth "an account of morality that is systematic, accessible, and usable"[35] for the discipline. The text drew attention for its attack on principlism (a term often thought to be a coinage of these authors) in general and Beauchamp and Childress' *Principles of Biomedical Ethics* in particular, which the authors describe as the "undeniably leading account" of the theory.[36]

While Gert, Culver, and Clouser refer to Beauchamp and Childress as "principlism's" "very best spokesmen,"[37] they do not actually provide any other examples of bioethics texts that adopt this approach, so it is difficult to determine what texts or thinkers they consider to be members of this "tradition." The criticism of Beauchamp and Childress' work in *Bioethics: A Return to Fundamentals* is a version of a more direct takedown of "principlism" that Clouser and Gert published in the *Journal of Medicine and Philosophy* in 1990, titled "A Critique of Principlism."[38] Curiously, however, Gert, Culver, and Clouser note that the fourth edition of Beauchamp and Childress' text was such a change from earlier versions that anything after this fourth edition no longer represents what Gert, Culver, and Clouser consider "principlism." They go on to say, somewhat oddly, that this actually strengthens their argument against the theory. That is, "it is not particularly Beauchamp and Childress that we are criticizing, but a paradigmatic form of principlism, which has been and still is thriving throughout the bioethical world."[39] It seems that only the earlier texts of the *Principles of Biomedical Ethics* are considered by Gert, Culver, and Clouser to represent this platonic form of principlism, which now exists only as a ghostly shadow text of Beauchamp and Childress' work.

Gert, Culver, and Clouser argue that while they have been referring to the approach expressed in *Principles of Biomedical Ethics* as a theory, "it is not in fact a theory, but rather a collection of 'principles,' which together are popularly mistakenly thought to function as a theory in guiding action."[40] For Gert, Culver, and Clouser, the principles in Beauchamp and Childress' text

> are really misnomers, since, when examined carefully, they are not action guides at all. Traditionally, principles really are action guides that summarize and encapsulate a whole theory and thus, in a shorthand manner, assist a moral agent in making a moral decision. Those kinds of principles are to be clearly distinguished from those of principlism. We argue that principles of principlism primarily function as checklists, naming issues worth remembering when one is considering a biomedical moral issue. "Consider this . . . Consider that . . . Remember to look for . . ." is what they tell the agent; they do not embody an articulated, established, and unified moral system capable of providing useful guidance.[41]

Gert, Culver, and Clouser imply here that principlism is not delivering on its promise: to guide actions according to one systematic moral theory. This summary is deceptive, however, for it profoundly misrepresents what principlism purports to be. There is no single, unified theory behind the principles, but Beauchamp and Childress never claimed there was; each principle derives from a variety of different theories. From the very first edition on, Beauchamp and Childress reject the goal of a "theory" as defined by Gert, Culver, and Clouser. Their aim is to provide a pragmatic movement beyond what at the time seemed like a fruitless battle between the theories (which *are* theories in Gert, Culver, and Clouser's sense of the word) of deontology and utilitarianism. As Beauchamp and Childress have often noted, they approached bioethics from different theoretical positions: Beauchamp is a utilitarian, Childress a deontologist. The principles of bioethics they advocate are justified by both of these theories, and thus principlism represents a pragmatic way to, in Rortian language, move the conversation in bioethics forward. The principles in *Principles of Biomedical Ethics* are never represented as action guides for a particular theory but rather mid-level principles justified by theories, plural. Indeed, another summary might characterize Beauchamp and Childress' principlism as a practical approach to resolving moral problems in bioethics, rather than as a failed "theory." In their response to Gert, Culver, and Clouser's critique, Beauchamp and Childress highlight this misrepresentation:

> We have not attempted a general ethical theory and do not claim that our principles mimic, are analogous to, or substitute for the foundational principles in leading classical theories such as utilitarianism (with its principle of utility) and Kantianism (with its categorical imperative).[42]

Engelhardt's *Foundations of Bioethics*, discussed earlier in relation to the concept of retrodiction, also engages Beauchamp and Childress' text, but interestingly only in its second edition. The first edition of Engelhardt's monograph was published in 1986, seven years after *Principles of Biomedical Ethics* was first published; Engelhardt's second edition of *The Foundations of Bioethics*, published in 1996, appeared two years after the *Principles of Biomedical Ethics*' fourth edition. This overlapping publication history is worth noting because of the important theoretical variations Beauchamp and Childress introduced in editions of the *Principles* over the years. When Engelhardt, in his second edition, distinguishes his two-principle approach from the four-principle approach advocated by Beauchamp and Childress, he cites the first edition of Beauchamp and Childress' book to draw the contrast.[43] Yet in doing this, he ignores the three subsequent editions in circulation—a choice that is most consequential in terms of the fourth edition, in which the authors had made changes to their theory that relate directly to the approach Engelhardt is seeking to promote.

Engelhardt's approach to bioethical controversies is nonfoundational, secular, and local. He justifies this approach by asserting the field's inability to arrive at a content-full ethic that can resolve moral problems. For him, there is no way to justify a moral position to someone who does not belong to the same moral community. In this respect, Engelhardt's worldview seems to entail a simple dichotomy between those within a particular circumscribed community and those outside of that community. D. Micah Hester refers to this argument as a form of "empty formalism," and calls its understanding of community "weak" in that Engelhardt seems to believe that community is only established within explicit contractual relationships.[44] For Engelhardt, the only thing a secular bioethics can provide is also the best that can be hoped for: a processual agreement that one will not force others (as one will, in turn, not be forced) to accept any particular medical intervention.

Engelhardt's summary of Beauchamp and Childress' approach reinforces his own premise that moral problems in bioethics are not soluble by a single theory. It also suggests that Beauchamp and Childress' goal is (like his) to establish a nonfoundationalist alternative to the fiction of an effective top-down approach.

> Beauchamp and Childress contend that middle-level principles can be used by individuals with different theoretical and moral perspectives, thus allowing both consequentialists and deontologists to employ the middle-level principles in order to resolve bioethical controversies. This tactic, if successful, would provide a nonfoundationalist approach to bioethics.[45]

The only problem with this summary is that in the fourth edition Engelhardt ignores that Beauchamp and Childress *do* propose a source for a content-full—but still nonfoundational—ethic: namely, the notion of "common morality," which provides an alternative schema to Engelhardt's simple dichotomy of stranger and friend.

Engelhardt's model of the moral world opines that nothing exists between friends and strangers that allows for an agreement (beyond the agreement not to force someone to follow another person's moral values without consent). Beauchamp and Childress' introduction of common morality into principlism, and in turn the need for Engelhardt to overlook this development in his summary, responds to a form of justification of decisions outside of any particular community. That is, regardless of whether one agrees to its actual existence, a common morality *is* a way to provide a nonfoundational approach to bioethics—which refutes Engelhardt's argument that no philosophical position can provide "content-full moral guidance unless one already fits them out with a particular moral substance."[46] The notion of common morality pushes against his claim by positing moral obligations that are not dependent upon any particular community's notion of the good. I am not suggesting that Engelhardt would concur on the existence of a common morality, of course. What I am saying is that his transformation of Beauchamp and Childress' text by drawing upon only the first edition permits him to dismiss their argument without taking on what would be a true challenge to his dichotomy between moral friends and moral strangers.

In "Zones of Consensus and Zones of Conflict: Questioning the 'Common Morality' Presumption in Bioethics," Leigh Turner takes up the very argument that Engelhardt skirts. Because Turner does not believe that universal moral values exist, he advocates for a morality based instead on pluralism. Pluralism responds to moral issues by acknowledging "the local, temporal character of 'moral worlds,'"[47] he writes, rather than clinging to some fairytale assumption of universally accepted values. While Turner focuses on the account of common morality provided in the fourth and later editions of the *Principles of Biomedical Ethics*, his essay is actually a broader attack on this notion of common morality—a notion espoused by theorists besides Beauchamp and Childress, including Gert, Culver, and Clouser. Turner zeroes in on Beauchamp and Childress' text rather than Gert, Culver, and Clouser's because, as he puts it, the *Principles of Biomedical Ethics* "played such an important role in setting the terms for debate within contemporary bioethics."[48]

Turner, at first glance, seems to present Beauchamp and Childress' argument through explicit intertextuality, that is, via the direct insertion of their text into his. For instance, he provides the reader with a generous quotation from the fifth edition of *Principles of Biomedical Ethics*:

> Since virtually everyone grows up with a basic understanding of the institution of morality, its norms are readily understood. All persons who are serious about living a moral life already grasp the core dimensions of morality. They know not to lie, not to steal property, to keep promises, to respect the rights of others, not to kill or cause harm to innocent persons, and the like. All persons serious about morality are comfortable with these rules and do not doubt their relevance and importance. . . . We will refer to the set of norms that all morally serious persons share as *the common morality*. The common morality contains moral norms that bind all persons in all places; no norms are more basic in the moral life. In recent years, the favored category to represent this universal core of morality in public discourse has been human rights, but moral obligation and moral virtue are no less vital parts of the common morality.[49]

Later, after also citing an essay Beauchamp published in 1999 on how his and Childress' principles "form the core of the common morality,"[50] Turner quotes extensively again from the fifth edition. Here is the passage Turner includes:

> Appeals to the common morality might also be *nonnormative*, or empirical, in which case they describe what all people believe. This thesis is more difficult

to defend and requires caution and qualification. It would be absurd to suppose that all persons do, in fact, accept the norms of the common morality. Many amoral, immoral, or selectively moral persons do not care about or identify with these or any other moral demands. Nonetheless, we believe that all persons in all cultures who are *serious about moral conduct* do accept the demands of the common morality.

Some readers will think that we are tripping over our own distinctions and begging the question by conflating the difference between *empirical claims* about what *is* universal in moral belief and *normative claims* about what *should be* universal in moral belief. Our formulation may seem to simply pack *our conception* of morality into the notion of morally serious persons, while failing to take seriously the empirical claims of multiculturalists. This criticism misunderstands our position. We accept the thesis that morality in the community-specific sense reflects significant cultural differences; but we think it is an institutional fact about morality, not merely our view of it, that it contains fundamental precepts. These fundamental precepts alone make it possible for persons to make cross-temporal and cross-cultural judgments and to assert firmly that not all practices in all cultural groups are morally acceptable.[51]

From this amount of direct quotation, the reader will likely conclude that Turner is being careful not to alter the meaning of Beauchamp and Childress' argument concerning common morality. Furthermore, these sections seem to demonstrate the validity of Turner's critique that a belief in common morality ignores the conflicting empirical evidence from history, anthropology, and sociology. Turner seems to be arguing that Beauchamp and Childress could make an argument for the existence of such a common morality—but only after they have done the hard work of exploring all available cross-cultural and transhistorical evidence for indications of such an entity. In response to Turner, Beauchamp's "A Defense of the Common Morality,"[52] counters that he has faith that when the empirical research is done, it will prove that they are correct in their assertion of these universal values. Yet Turner believes that the evidence is already in. Beauchamp's "Defense" has a more powerful response to Turner's argument, however: Beauchamp expresses puzzlement that Turner overlooks the distinction Beauchamp and Childress make between "common morality" and "particular moralities"[53]—a distinction that acknowledges pluralism but at the same time promotes the existence of universal principles.

Genette considers *excision*, or taking parts out of the hypotext, a form of intertextual hypertextuality; that is, it involves direct quotation of the hypotext, but only of certain selections.[54] Genette is concerned mainly with global versions of excision, such as the common excision of the third and fourth journeys from Jonathan Swift's *Gulliver's Travels*, which leaves only Gulliver's adventures in Lilliput and Brobdingnag. Genette calls this type of excision *amputation*, entailing "a single massive excision"[55] of a text. The other form Genette identifies is *trimming*, or pruning, by removing smaller sections of the hypotext. Turner's account of Beauchamp and Childress' concept of common morality is an example of the latter. Between his first and second quoted passages, Beauchamp and Childress include an entire paragraph dedicated to the very distinction. The paragraph he omits, but which immediately follows his first direct quotation, concerns Beauchamp and Childress' definition of common morality:

> Morality consists of more than the common morality, and we should never confuse or conflate the two. For example, morality includes moral ideals that individuals and groups voluntarily accept, communal norms that bind only members of specific moral communities, extraordinary virtues, and the like. The common morality, by contrast, comprises all and only those norms that all morally serious persons accept as authoritative. Here two distinctions are crucial: The first is between "morality" in the universal sense and "morality" in a community-specific sense; and the second is between nonnormative (that is, empirical) claims about what is universal in moral belief and normative claims about what should be universal in moral belief. These distinctions are indispensable for understanding this book's assumptions and arguments.[56]

Turner trims out the section in his presentation of Beauchamp and Childress' argument, and for good reason. Here, the authors acknowledge the exact form of pluralism that Turner claims they do not feel the need to respond to. In short, Turner's representation of Beauchamp and Childress' account of common morality appears at first to be simply a series of intertextual quotations, that is, lacking any form of transformation. Through excision, however, he presents their argument as if it does not make any distinction between particular communal morality, which they argue is "nonnormative" and "empirical," and their common morality, which is normative and universal. Notably, Beauchamp's assertion that he is confused that Turner "altogether rejects" this distinction is also not accurate, for Turner's trimming makes rejection unnecessary: he simply removes its existence as something to which his argument needs to respond.

Rosamund Rhodes confronts the notion of a common morality head-on. In *The Trusted Doctor: Medical Ethics and Professionalism*, Rhodes advocates provocatively for a medical ethics based on an "uncommon morality account." Rhodes believes that the moral obligations for physicians are internal to the profession, inherently distinct from the obligations and values of those outside the profession. As Rhodes states, she wishes to replace medical ethics based on common morality, including Beauchamp and Childress' approach, with a "contractarian constructivism" that acknowledges the distinctive and unique character of the morality of the medical profession.

Rhodes is quite explicit that an attack on common morality is an essential element of her work. Persuading readers to reject common morality

> is critically important because if I can show that the principles or rules of common morality are inadequate guides for the action of medical professionals, and that in some circumstances they direct doctors to do what good doctors should not do, that demonstration would prove that common morality accounts of medical ethics are inadequate.[57]

In fact, in comparing "everyday ethics" with medical ethics, Rhodes concludes that the two are not only distinct but even "incompatible."[58]

That is not the way Beauchamp and Childress see it, according to Rhodes. In her words, Beauchamp and Childress' argument for a medical ethic based on common morality assumes that "professional ethics is nothing more than narrowly specified conclusions from common morality."[59] To her, Beauchamp and Childress consider medical ethics simply "an extrapolation of the principles of common morality."[60] Yet Beauchamp and Childress cannot maintain this claim in light of all the moral obligations expected of physicians, she says, which demonstrates the invalidity of their argument; Beauchamp and Childress must acknowledge that physicians have special roles and duties beyond those specified by common morality.

Rhodes' summary of Beauchamp and Childress portrays their ideal relationship between common morality and biomedical ethics as a simple extension. A more accurate representation would have medical professional ethics as one of several subsets (unique professional ethics) within a broader domain (common morality). This sense of the larger purview of the common morality is illustrated when Beauchamp and Childress write that the values from within a particular realm, such as that of medicine, "are not morally justified if they violate norms in the common morality."[61] It is reinforced by Beauchamp and Childress' attention to issues of resource allocation and research ethics—matters that only indirectly concern physicians, but which certainly fall within biomedical ethics. In other words, *Principles of Biomedical Ethics* seeks to provide the ethical foundations for addressing issues that include, but reach well beyond, the issues facing physicians. To characterize Beauchamp and Childress' argument as ignoring the unique obligations of physicians is thus a misrepresentation—a misrepresentation that allows Rhodes to create space for a new ethic that is unique to medical professionals and is radically separate from the common morality.

In *Community as Healing*, D. Micah Hester argues for a bioethics that is based on American pragmatism, particularly the pragmatism of John Dewey. Before fully developing his theoretical position, Hester, in chapter two of the book, notes that he will not attempt to address all the prior theoretical positions developed in bioethics but instead will "look at what is still quite possibly the most influential approach to contemporary bioethics: the use of basic bioethics principles."[62] The two texts Hester examines in detail are Beauchamp and Childress' *Principles of Biomedical Ethics* and Engelhardt's *Foundations of Bioethics*. In his summary of Beauchamp and Childress, Hester is very cognizant that their argument has changed from the first edition to the current version at the time (the fourth edition), but he argues that their approach's essential core—the four principles—remains the same.

Hester's summary focuses primarily on a section titled "Coherentism" in Beauchamp and Childress' fourth edition, which Hester puts in his own section titled "The Theory." Coherentism, according to Beauchamp and Childress, is an alternative to both "top-down" approaches (as principlism was often initially criticized for) and "bottom-up" approaches, for it is a moral theory that "moves in both directions."[63] Hester explains that this approach, which draws upon the work of John Rawls, begins with "considered judgments" and then moves into "reflexive equilibrium." Hester goes on to characterize Beauchamp and Childress' principles as "a rational reconstruction of our considered judgments," but notes that "the considered judgments may, through a reflection on the implications of the principles, be changed in order to comply more closely with the principles themselves."[64] At this point in his summary, Hester observes that at first glance, a pragmatist like himself might detect in this theory a Dewey-like emphasis on a moral theory that is process-oriented, enabling "a movement from experience to theory and a movement back to experience with adjustments at both ends."[65] But the similarity is not earned, Hester says. Their theory does not truly embody that back and forth movement, and the promise of moving beyond inductivism and deductivism is never fulfilled.

> Beauchamp and Childress's language betrays them when they speak of the activities of "reflective equilibrium" that starts not at the level of particular experiences and judgments but at the level of "paradigm" judgments (judgment already abstracted from particular experiences). From there considered judgments are items "matched and pruned" in order to "render [them] coherent with premises of theory" and *not* vice versa. They speak most pointedly to the "second movement" down from ethical theory, adjusting considered judgment to principles, but not principles to judgments.[66]

This lack of even processual movement of bottom influencing top is what prompts Hester to propose a truly Dewey-like pragmatism as his foundation for bioethics.

A notable absence from Hester's summary, however, is Beauchamp and Childress' discussion of what they call "wide reflective equilibrium," which they state "occurs when we evaluate the strengths and weaknesses of all plausible moral judgments, principles, and relevant ground theories."[67] In other words, Beauchamp and Childress argue that principles are themselves proper subjects of "pruning, adjusting, and rendering coherent"—not just the judgments made on particular cases. Not including this final part of the discussion is necessary for Hester's argument, for including it would reveal that pragmatism, at least in its promotion of reflective movement between concrete experience and abstract principles, has nothing new to add to principlism.

One final example of how summary enables the authors of foundational texts to make room for their theory is more of an anti-example. Richard Zaner's essay "Experience and Moral Life: A Phenomenological Approach to Bioethics,"[68] was published in an anthology titled *A Matter of Principles: Ferment in U.S. Bioethics*.[69] As its title suggests, the anthology was focused on presentations and criticisms of principlism. In their introduction, the editors note that bioethics approaches that use "moral principles to address issues and resolve case quandaries" have become the predominant theoretical position in the United States,[70] and their two "major" examples of principlism are Veatch's *Theory of Medical Ethics* and Engelhardt's *Foundations of Bioethics*. The most influential example of this position, however, is Beauchamp and Childress' *Principles of Biomedical Ethics*, which the editors characterize as "a virtual bible to some practitioners."

Most of the contributors follow the editors in addressing their critique to one or more of these three texts. Zaner, on the other hand, refuses to respond to Beauchamp and Childress' text (or any other principlist text); he dismisses all texts that use this approach. He begins with the bald statement: "This essay veers away from the prevailing view in biomedical ethics: the applied, or principlist, view."[71] Providing no account of Beauchamp and Childress' text, Zaner argues that

> [a]s it seems untoward to introduce a Grand Duchess to assembled personages too early in the evening, so does it seem premature to address such grand issues as "principles" at a time when ethical deliberation within clinical life has only just begun.[72]

Zaner defends this lack of attention to the very subject of the anthology by arguing that principles cannot precede a phenomenological examination of the clinical setting in which moral issues arise (which is to say, his particular theory). This approach is somewhat akin to what Harold Bloom, in his "map of misreading," refers to as *kenosis*, in which a writer breaks from a powerful precursor by emptying their own status and thus also empties out the precursor;[73] Zaner's refusal to summarize the principlists' view drains these dominant voices of their importance. The Grand Duchess may enter the room at some point—and we may want her there—but the room is not yet ready.

I do not wish, however, to make it seem that Beauchamp and Childress are in some manner simply victims of hypertextuality, for the need to summarize and respond to other works, as noted above, is simply an essential part of all academic discourse. As already discussed, one of Beauchamp and Childress' most notable critics was Clouser and Gert; Beauchamp and Childress refer to them as their "most unsparing critics."[74] In a subsequent edition of *Principles of Biomedical Ethics*, Beauchamp and Childress respond to Clouser and Gert. In one section of their response, Beauchamp and Childress challenge the criticism "that the principle of beneficence expresses a moral ideal, not a moral obligation"[75] as is asserted in principlism. Since Clouser and Gert contend that there is no moral duty to either promote good or prevent evil, if one were able to demonstrate that they do not follow their own assertion that there is only a universal moral duty to not cause harm, one would show an inconsistency in the argument. Beauchamp and Childress do so by looking at a general account of moral duties that Gert makes in his book *Morality: Its Nature and Justification*. They note that in this argument Gert includes in his basic moral rules the "obligations of beneficence."[76] They then quote Gert's own explanation concerning such a duty. Here are the first two sentences of their quotation: "Although duties, in general, go with offices, jobs, roles, etc., there are some duties that seem more general. . . . In any civilized society, if a child collapses in your arms, you have a duty to seek help."[77] The ellipses in the quote are an example of *Genette's* excision. If one looks at the original source, one will see that the amount of material that Beauchamp and Childress have removed between sentence one and sentence two is substantial—so substantial, three entire paragraphs—that if added, it would far exceed fair use for intertextuality. What they have removed from Gert's text in this quote includes an extensive discussion of how generally people speak of duties in a manner that actually means "you ought." Gert explains that in his argument duty has a far more limited meaning in that it only pertains "because of some special circumstances."[78] After quoting the sentence concerning the duty in "any civilized society" to take care of a child that "collapses in your arms," Beauchamp and Childress then elide the rest of the paragraph and begin quoting the next paragraph that begins: "In most civilized societies one has a duty to help . . ." What is particularly notable is that Beauchamp and Childress do not provide an explicit noting of an ellipsis between the sentence that concerns the duty to help a child and the duty in "most civilized societies," for Gert concludes his discussion of this obligation to help the child by stating, "This duty cannot simply be called the duty to aid those in distress, for we do not have a duty to send money to those who are starving. It is, of course, morally good to do this, but we have no duty to be morally good."[79] Gert makes a clear distinction between an act that he thinks may be considered morally good and an act for which one has a moral duty to accomplish, and he does not believe that one has a universal moral duty to help others. Beauchamp and Childress have, in their quotation of Gert, taken out the aspects of his argument that would counter their claim that he asserts in his moral duties one to do good for others.

CONCLUSION

This chapter has looked at two basic forms of transformation in bioethics texts: continuation and summary. The first describes how bioethicists developed their approaches by extending prior moral theories into the subject of health care. The second identifies the various methods by which a prior hypotext, which is in some manner in agonic struggle with the new text, must be reproduced but also reduced. Without a reduction, the hypertext would be forced to comprise in full all of its intertexts—so that every text would be akin to the map in Lewis Carroll's *Sylvie and Bruno Concluded*, in which the map has "the scale of mile to the mile," making the map and that which it is mapping exactly the same size. The character relating the existence of this map notes that now they "use the country itself, as its own map."[80] Reduction is inevitable in academic discourse, but as Genette reminds us, "One cannot reduce a text without diminishing it or, more precisely, without subtracting from it some part or parts."[81] The various summaries of Beauchamp and Childress' *Principles of Biomedical Ethics* examined above show how these hypertextual accounts should be viewed as rhetorical acts, redescriptions that allow the new text to show a deficiency in the prior text.

I do not wish to suggest that the various criticisms of and new methods proposed in response to Beauchamp and Childress' theory are not valid—only that their redescription and subtractions often weaken their opponent. If my own account is accepted as valid, though, it does raise the question of intentionality. Should we assume that these manipulations represent an unconscious misprision of the prior work, as Bloom might say? Or are they what Ralph Waldo Emerson describes in his essay "The Poet" as *miswritings*? The degree by which the summary is described accurately matters little because the consequences for the reader are the same; in each instance, the hypotext is rewritten in order to strengthen the argument within the hypertext. Summaries become, in bioethics rhetorical devices, for in their choices of what to include and what to leave out, they redescribe their predecessors in a manner that creates space for their new insights. As Borges once observed, "The fact is that every writer *creates* his own precursors. His work modifies our conception of the past, as it will modify the future."[82]

NOTES

1. Andrew Jameston and Albert R. Jonsen, "America, Bioethics in," in *Bioethics*, ed. Bruce Jennings (Farmington Hills, MI: Macmillan Reference, Gale, Cengage Learning, 2014), 196.

2. Robert Veatch, *Theory of Medical Ethics* (New York: Basic Books, 1981), 3.

3. Roland Barthes, "From Work to Text," in *Image Music Text, trans. Stephen Heath*(New York: Farrar, Straus and Giroux, 1977), 160.

4. Gérard Genette, *Palimpsests: Literature in the Second Degree*, trans. Channa Newman and Claude Doubinsky (Lincoln, NE: University of Nebraska Press, 1997), 1.

5. Genette, *Palimpsests: Literature in the Second Degree*, 1.

6. It should be noted that, as already mentioned, the concept of "intertextuality" already had a relatively clear meaning as used in literary criticism, and Genette acknowledges himself that using the term to mean a particular type of what is usually called intertextuality causes confusion. In order to remain consistent for this chapter, I will be using Genette's definition of intertextuality and will use his term transtextuality to refer to what intertextuality is more commonly used for. See Genette, *Palimpsests: Literature in the Second Degree*, 1–2.

7. Genette, *Palimpsests: Literature in the Second Degree*, 4.

8. Genette, *Palimpsests: Literature in the Second Degree*, 6.

9. Genette, *Palimpsests: Literature in the Second Degree*, 175.

10. Genette, *Palimpsests: Literature in the Second Degree*, 6, 181.

11. Genette, *Palimpsests: Literature in the Second Degree*, 177.

12. Genette, *Palimpsests: Literature in the Second Degree*, 175.

13. Italics in original Norman Daniels, *Just Health Care*, Studies in Philosophy and Health Policy (Cambridge; New York: Cambridge University Press, 1985), 43.

14. Drew Leder, *The Distressed Body: Rethinking Illness, Imprisonment, and Healing* (Chicago IL: University of Chicago Press, 2016), 107.

15. Griffin Trotter, *The Loyal Physician: Roycean Ethics and the Practice of Medicine* (Nashville, TN: Vanderbilt University Press, 1997), 12.

16. Judith Andre, *Bioethics as Practice* (Chapel Hill, NC: University of North Carolina Press, 2002), 50.

17. Andre, *Bioethics as Practice*, 50.

18. Laurie Zoloth, *Health Care and the Ethics of Encounter: A Jewish Discussion of Social Justice* (Chapel Hill, NC: University of North Carolina Press, 1999), xi–xii.

19. Leder, *The Distressed Body: Rethinking Illness, Imprisonment, and Healing*, 109.

20. Genette, *Palimpsests: Literature in the Second Degree*, 238–251.

21. Thomas Tomlinson, *Methods in Medical Ethics: Critical Perspectives* (Oxford: Oxford University Press, 2012), xvi.

22. Robert Stam, "Beyond Fidelity: The Dialogics of Adaptation," *Film Adaptation* (2000): 54–76.

23. See Tod Chambers, *The Fiction of Bioethics* (New York: Routledge, 1999).

24. Tom Koch, "The Hippocratic Thorn in Bioethics' Hide: Cults, Sects, and Strangeness," *Journal of Medicine and Philosophy* 39, no. 1 (February 2014): 86.

25. Genette, *Palimpsests: Literature in the Second Degree*, 251.

26. Margaret Urban Walker, *Moral Understandings: A Feminist Study in Ethics* (New York: Routledge, 1998), 7–9.
27. Edmund Pincoffs, "Quandary Ethics," *Mind* 80, no. 320 (1971): 552–571.
28. Leigh Turner, "Medical Facilities as Moral Worlds," *Medical Humanities* 28, no. 1 (2002): 19–22.
29. Hilde Lindemann Nelson, "Four Narrative Approaches to Bioethics," in *Handbook of Bioethics* (New York: Kluwer Academic Publshers, 2004), 163; Howard Brody, *Stories of Sickness*, 2nd ed. (Oxford: Oxford University Press, 2003), 176–177.
30. Richard B. Davis, "The Principlism Debate: A Critical Overview," *The Journal of Medicine and Philosophy* 20, no. 1 (1995): 85.
31. John Hyde Evans, "A Sociological Account of the Growth of Principlism," *Hastings Center Report* 30, no. 5 (September–October 2000): 31–38.
32. John D. Arras, "The Hedgehog and the Borg: Common Morality in Bioethics," *Theoretical Medicine and Bioethics* 30 (2009): 12.
33. Bernard Gert, Charles M. Culver, and K. Danner Clouser, *Bioethics: A Systematic Approach*, 2nd ed. (New York: Oxford University Press, 2006), viii.
34. Charles M. Culver and Bernard Gert, *Philosophy in Medicine: Conceptual and Ethical Issues in Medicine and Psychiatry* (New York: Oxford University Press, 1982).
35. Bernard Gert, Charles M. Culver, and K. Danner Clouser, *Bioethics: A Return to Fundamentals* (New York: Oxford University Press, 1997), 1.
36. Gert, Culver, and Clouser, *Bioethics: A Return to Fundamentals*, 72.
37. Gert, Culver, and Clouser, *Bioethics: A Return to Fundamentals*, 72.
38. K. Danner Clouser and Bernard Gert, "A Critique of Principlism," *The Journal of Medicine and Philosophy* 15, no. 2 (1990): 219–236.
39. Gert, Culver, and Clouser, *Bioethics: A Return to Fundamentals*, 72.
40. Gert, Culver, and Clouser, *Bioethics: A Return to Fundamentals*, 74.
41. Gert, Culver, and Clouser, *Bioethics: A Return to Fundamentals*, 75.
42. Tom L. Beauchamp and James F. Childress, *Principles of Biomedical Ethics*, 4th ed. (New York: Oxford University Press, 1994), 106.
43. H. Tristram Engelhardt, *The Foundations of Bioethics*, 2nd ed. (New York: Oxford University Press, 1996), 90, footnote 47.
44. D. Micah Hester, *Community as Healing: Pragmatist Ethics in Medical Encounters* (Lanham, MD: Rowman & Littlefield, 2001), 32.
45. Engelhardt, *The Foundations of Bioethics*, 56.
46. Engelhardt, *The Foundations of Bioethics*, 58.
47. Leigh Turner, "Zones of Consensus and Zones of Conflict: Questioning the 'Common Morality' Presumption in Bioethics," *Kennedy Institute of Ethics Journal* 13, no. 3 (2003): 206.
48. Turner, "Zones of Consensus and Zones of Conflict: Questioning the 'Common Morality' Presumption in Bioethics," 196.
49. As quoted in Turner, "Zones of Consensus and Zones of Conflict: Questioning the 'Common Morality' Presumption in Bioethics," 199–200.
50. As quoted Turner, "Zones of Consensus and Zones of Conflict: Questioning the 'Common Morality' Presumption in Bioethics," 200.
51. As quoted Turner, "Zones of Consensus and Zones of Conflict: Questioning the 'Common Morality' Presumption in Bioethics," 200.

52. Tom L. Beauchamp, "A Defense of the Common Morality," *Kennedy Institute of Ethics Journal* 13, no. 3 (2003): 259–274.

53. Beauchamp, "A Defense of the Common Morality," 263.

54. Genette, *Palimpsests: Literature in the Second Degree*, 229–235.

55. Genette, *Palimpsests: Literature in the Second Degree*, 229.

56. Tom L. Beauchamp and James F. Childress, *Principles of Biomedical Ethics*, 5th ed. (New York: Oxford University Press, 2001), 3.

57. Rosamond Rhodes, *The Trusted Doctor: Medical Ethics and Professionalism* (New York: Oxford University Press, 2020), 14.

58. Rhodes, *The Trusted Doctor: Medical Ethics and Professionalism*, 13.

59. Rhodes, *The Trusted Doctor: Medical Ethics and Professionalism*, 21.

60. Rhodes, *The Trusted Doctor: Medical Ethics and Professionalism*, 346.

61. Beauchamp and Childress, *Principles of Biomedical Ethics*, 7th ed. 5.

62. Hester, *Community as Healing: Pragmatist Ethics in Medical Encounters*, 21.

63. Beauchamp and Childress, *Principles of Biomedical Ethics*, 20.

64. Hester, *Community as Healing: Pragmatist Ethics in Medical Encounters*, 23.

65. Hester, *Community as Healing: Pragmatist Ethics in Medical Encounters*, 24.

66. Hester, *Community as Healing: Pragmatist Ethics in Medical Encounters*, 24.

67. Beauchamp and Childress, *Principles of Biomedical Ethics*, 22.

68. Richard M. Zaner, "Experience and Moral Life: A Phenomenological Approach to Bioethics," in *A Matter of Principles?: Ferment in U.S. Bioethics*, ed. E. R. DuBose, R. P. Hamel, and L. J. O'Connell (Valley Forge, PA: Trinity, 1994) 211–239.

69. Edwin R. DuBose, Ronald P. Hamel, and Laurence J. O'Connell, eds., *A Matter of Principles?: Ferment in U.S. Bioethics* (Valley Forge, PA: Trinity Press International, 1994).

70. Edwin R. DuBose, Ronald P. Hamel, and Laurence J. O'Connell, "Introduction," in *A Matter of Principles?: Ferment in U.S. Bioethics*, ed. E. R. DuBose, R. P. Hamel, and L. J. O'Connell (Valley Forge, PA: Trinity, 1994), 1.

71. Zaner, "Experience and Moral Life: A Phenomenological Approach to Bioethics," 211.

72. Zaner, "Experience and Moral Life: A Phenomenological Approach to Bioethics," 211.

73. Harold Bloom, *The Anxiety of Influence: A Theory of Poetry*, 2nd ed. (New York: Oxford University Press, 1997), 77–92.

74. Tom L. Beauchamp and James F. Childress, *Principles of Biomedical Ethics* (New York: Oxford University Press, 2019), 428.

75. Beauchamp and Childress, *Principles of Biomedical Ethics*, 431.

76. Beauchamp and Childress, *Principles of Biomedical Ethics*, 431.

77. As quoted in Beauchamp and Childress, *Principles of Biomedical Ethics*, 431.

78. Bernard Gert and Bernard Gert, *Morality: A New Justification of the Moral Rules* (New York: Oxford University Press, 1988), 154.

79. Gert and Gert, *Morality: A New Justification of the Moral Rules*, 155.

80. Lewis Carroll, *Sylvie and Bruno Concluded* (London: MacMillan, 1895), 169.

81. Genette, *Palimpsests: Literature in the Second Degree*, 229.

82. Jorge Luis Borges, "Kafka and His Precursors," in *Labyrinths* (New York: New Directions, 1964), 201.

Conclusion

The Bioethicist as Poet

Judith Jarvis Thomson's abortion thought experiment asks the reader to imagine waking up one morning attached to a famous violinist who will be using your kidneys for nine months in order to recover from an illness. After this period of time, the violinist will have recovered, freeing you once again to live your life. Thomson closes out this thought experiment by echoing the language of those who oppose abortion on the grounds that it entails the murder of another person. She has the director of her imagined hospital, who had initially assured you that he had no knowledge of the actions taken by the Society of Music Lovers (the group responsible for attaching the violinist to your kidneys), agree that the whole thing is "tough luck"—but then conclude,

> All persons have a right to life, and violinists are persons. Granted you have a right to decide what happens in and to your body, but a person's right to life outweighs your right to decide what happens in and to your body. So you cannot ever be unplugged from him.[1]

Then Thomson returns to the argument in her own voice, observing that we would, of course, find the hospital director's statement "outrageous."

As discussed earlier, this thought experiment was created by Thomson to dissociate the issue of abortion from the question of when life begins or what counts as personhood. The dissociation is accomplished by *redescription*: Thomson's novel thought experiment provides a new context for evaluating the moral duty of a person who is pregnant. In his well-known response to Thomson's essay, "Nature as Demonic in Thomson's Defense of Abortion," John T. Wilcox attacks what he believes is the central ingredient of her argument, that is, it "is basically an argument by analogy."[2] Throughout his essay, Wilcox challenges the validity of comparing abortion to this fantastical scenario, at one time complaining that "the violinist example is *weird*."[3] Wilcox's response is, to some degree, itself "weird," in that it seems to express genuine concern that readers will think Thomson's scenario either *has* happened or that it is medically plausible. For most readers, I suspect, Thomson's violinist is a case rooted firmly in science fiction.[4] But I think Wilcox is correct in seeing the essay as built around Thomson's belief that the answer to this thought experiment is self-evident: we might think it admirable if someone would agree to stay attached to the violinist, but we would never say that it would be the *right* of the violinist—who is inarguably a "human life" and a "person"—to demand the use of the body of another person, even if it were for a specific period of time.

With this thought experiment, Thomson is creating what I contend is a new *context* for the abortion debate. The origin of the word "text" is from the Latin *texere*, which means to weave or join. The word "context" combines *texere* with *con*, which means "together." The word's origin suggests that when we refer to context, we are talking about when one text is woven together with another. But what counts as a text, and who does the weaving? The literary critic Jonathan Culler addresses these concerns in his analysis of the famous debate between the philosophers Jacques Derrida and John Searle, who disagreed as to whether John Austin's notion of speech acts extended beyond "serious," intentional speech acts to cover "non-serious" or fictional utterances. While some have argued that the audience will determine the validity, and thus the social force, of any particular speech act, Culler sees a problem with that assumption. As he argues, "There is no limit in principle to what might be included in a given context, to what might be shown to be relevant to the performance of a particular speech act."[5] Or to put it simply, "context is boundless." When we enter a text, the author has already decided which texts will be woven together to generate that encounter—and there is immense rhetorical power in those decisions.

Consider the number of other ways in which the abortion debate has been contextualized, for example. With each new text, the act of terminating a pregnancy can be redescribed as a matter of social standing, science, common sense, religion, and so on.

Take Sydney Callahan's essay against abortion, "Abortion and the Sexual Agenda." Callahan describes pregnancy in a manner that denies thinking through analogies. She asserts that, unlike medical activities such as organ transplants, contraception, or mastectomies, pregnancy is not simply an issue (as it has been framed by some) of a right to control one's body, for during a pregnancy, "another body will emerge. One's own body no longer exists as a single unit but is engendering another organism's life. This dynamic passage from conception to birth is genetically ordered and universally found in the human species."[6] Callahan rejects attempting to describe pregnancy through other medical conditions or "strained philosophical analogies," including those that concern famous violinists. Callahan, in this essay, goes on to stake out what she calls a feminist pro-life position, as opposed to the typical alignment of feminists as pro-choice. As she argues, the advocacy for the "rights and liberation" of women "are pragmatically linked to fetal rights because to obtain true equality, women need (1) more social support and changes in the structure of society, and (2) increased self-confidence, self-expectations, and self-esteem." Without providing adequate support for women, our society perpetuates "our devastating feminization of poverty."[7] For Callahan, if we argue that the decision to end a pregnancy is solely within the purview of the woman, then why should men have any obligation to assume responsibility in raising children? Callahan's argument hinges on describing the morality of abortion as linked to women's status in society—just not in the way pro-choice feminists have claimed. It is for this reason that labeling her argument as feminist is so important to the argument; Callahan justifies her distinctive position on the abortion debate by recontextualizing "fetal rights" as aligned with a resistance to, rather than an extension of, women's oppression.

A different context for the abortion debate can be found in Gregg Easterbrook's essay "Abortion and Brain Waves." For Easterbrook, the most relevant context is not the pregnant woman's body or the status of the fetus in terms of personhood, but our understanding of the human brain. Easterbrook states that research into the development of the brain of a fetus reveals information that "neither side" of the abortion debate "wants to hear."[8] Describing this research as a matter of "cold-hearted chemistry," Easterbrook argues that

> It is time to admit what everyone knows and what the new science makes clear: that third-trimester abortion should be very tightly restricted. The hopelessly confusing viability standard should be dropped in favor of a bright line drawn at the start of the third trimester, when complex fetal brain activity begins.[9]

Charles Gardner's "Is an Embryo a Person?" also contextualizes abortion vis a vis science texts. Gardner begins his essay by noting that the abortion debate has been focused on "women's rights" versus "babies' rights," but the question that must first be addressed is for him a biological one: *what is the embryo*? He charts how anti-abortion advocates have "increasingly used" a "biological argument" to support their position, which he feels is at its core a religious argument. "This purportedly scientific argument comes as a surprise to embryologists, however, for it contradicts all that they have learned in the past few decades."[10] Like Easterbrook, Gardner asserts that once the debate is placed within the correct, scientific context, the position one should take on abortion becomes obvious. For Gardner, the pro-life position and the pro-choice one both have "blind spots." For the pro-life advocates, they refuse to acknowledge the issues of women's health and personal freedom. For the pro-choice, this blind spot resides in not attending to what we now know about the brain development of the fetus. He states baldly,

> [i]t is time to admit what everyone knows and what the new science makes clear: that third-trimester abortion should very tightly restricted. The hopelessly confusing viability standard should be dropped in favor of a bright line drawn at the start of the third trimester, when complex fetal brain activity begins.[11]

In her book *The Scarlet A*, Katie Watson shifts the setting of the debate, describing abortion not in terms of the research lab but instead in terms of the clinical encounter. In particular, Watson argues that our understanding of abortion in the United States needs to take into account its "ordinariness." As she notes, abortions "are safe, routine medical procedures. Conceptually speaking, they are consistent with the goals of medicine: at a patient's request, a physician brings the patient's body back to its baseline state."[12] While Watson acknowledges that a pregnancy is not an "illness," she describes it as fitting comfortably within the ordinary activities of a clinical setting.[13] Watson argues that

> [w]hether a patient is unhappy about a broken leg, a lung infection, or an unwanted pregnancy, in ordinary medicine, a patient tells a doctor he or she doesn't want the health risks and life-altering effects of a change in his or her body, and the doctor uses a drug or procedure to bring the body back to the way it was.[14]

While Watson concedes that pointing out that something is common does not mean it is justified, she believes that the fact it has become a common part of clinical care "raises a question of moral intuition": while parts of our society continue to engage in a debate over the morality of abortion, "Americans' behavior has quietly established abortion as routine medical care."[15] For Watson, this redescription of abortion should result in seeing the practice in its proper context: as a regular part of ordinary health care.

Philip Ivanhoe introduces two new contexts for the abortion debate. In "A Confucian Perspective on Abortion," Ivanhoe argues that a Confucian perspective means considering abortion in light of the family and a reverence for life—and in light of the pregnant woman as a "fellow human being and member of the community." The issue of abortion can only be resolved by attempting to harmonize these concerns. Ultimately, he writes, once abortion is viewed within the context of a rich understanding of family that includes notions of "parental love, filial piety, and brotherly love," the notion of "abortion on demand" must be rejected.[16] Ivanhoe points out that this notion of reverence for life in a Confucian view is different from the Western conception of a "right to life," for it is not justified on the basis of individualism but on the interrelated web of human life.

Another form of context employed in the abortion debate could be characterized as temporal. In *Every Third Woman in America: How Legal Abortion Transformed Our Nation*, for example, David Grimes bases an argument for the legalization of abortion in the United States on the historical context of the number of lives lost when it was illegal.[17] Gary Leber, on the other hand, links abortion to a different past in his essay titled "We Must Rescue Them."

> It will not do to complain that there is a worldwide consensus that something like Nazi Germany must not happen again or that we are too civilized to let it happen. In this country alone, we've already destroyed *four times* the number of people that Hitler did.[18]

Finally, in the oft-cited "Why Abortion is Immoral," Don Marquis argues that the best temporal context for understanding the impact of abortion is not with respect to the past, but to the future: the fetus' relationship to future experiences, a future biography.[19]

Albert Jonsen and Stephen Toulmin's classic text, *The Abuse of Casuistry*, is framed around the abortion debate. After their book-length argument for a revival of casuistry, they return at last to abortion, to show how this intractable problem becomes tractable when attended to in terms of particular "cases." The context for their discussion is the "rhetorical extremes" of the positions of the pro-life and pro-choice movements, so that the real problem becomes the tendency that

> [o]nly people whose minds are too firmly made up to reconsider the complexities of the abortion issue can say in advance that none of these changes [in the development of the fetus over the time of a pregnancy] has any possible relevance to the matter.[20]

Noting that the traditional Catholic thinking on abortion did, in fact, take these differences into account, Jonsen and Toulmin diagnose the true problem in the abortion debate as extremism in the contemporary American political context.

In each of these descriptions of abortion, a host of different texts is related to abortion. If context is boundless, as Culler suggests, then we can interpret a text against anything in the entire world—an insight staked by the literary school of New Historicism, which focused on the "historicity of texts and the textuality of history."[21] Yet within a single text, as seen in the examples above, context is also inherently constrained, in that particular texts are woven together with other texts by the author. The reader could link the argument to texts outside the "work" being read, of course, but authors always, to some degree, get to create their own context.

The concept of context has been important to bioethics, and for some, seeing moral issues in relation to a particular context is the discipline's defining feature, as it is to all forms of applied ethics. Indeed, the necessity of attending to context can be found in almost all bioethical schools and methods. In advocating for a phenomenological approach, Richard Zaner argues that a key virtue is that phenomenology presents moral problems "solely within the contexts of their actual occurrence."[22] Alisa Carse characterizes a care ethics approach to bioethics as "contextual rather than abstract."[23] Joseph Fins and Franklin Miller argue for their particular form of clinical pragmatism by noting how it entails "a contextually situated analysis."[24] Micah Hester in *Community as Healing* also draws upon the pragmatists, proclaiming that "any appropriate ethical principle must arise out of the context if it is to have any meaning to the given situation."[25] In *Stories of Sickness* Howard Brody argues that one of the appeals of a narrative approach to ethics is that it allows one to judge the situation "within the context of a person's life story,"[26] and Larry Churchill states simply, in his famous "Hermeneutics of Consent Forms," that "context is everything."[27] Even Tom Beauchamp and James Childress, the preeminent voices for a principles-based approach to bioethics, affirm that "practical moral problems often require that we make our general norms specific for a particular context or range of cases."[28]

In *No Longer Patient*, Susan Sherwin refers to this abiding concern as "the pursuit of context in bioethics." Sherwin concludes her historical survey of this tendency by observing, "we can see that the trend in medical ethics has been to examine moral issues in context and to avoid dependence on general, abstract rules and rights."[29] Margaret Urban Walker remarks on the problematic nature of this fealty to context, however, because we lack "a sufficient guide without some theoretical guidance about which features of context are ripe with possibilities for supporting or compromising moral values." As she goes on to ask bluntly, how exactly do we determine which things qualify as "morally relevant context"?[30]

It has been the argument of this book that the answer to this question is quite simple: the relevant context is whatever texts the author has chosen to weave together, and those texts will almost always be ones that offer rhetorical support for the argument being made. Bioethics arguments always entail some description of the world in which the moral theories and positions are applied. The history of bioethics is, thus, very much a history of redescription.

BIOETHICS AND STRONG POETS

As I noted in the introduction, I borrow the concept of redescription from Richard Rorty, who explicates it in his book *Contingency, Irony, and Solidarity*. In his radical revision of what philosophers do (and, more importantly, what he *thinks* they should do), Rorty says that philosophy is most useful when it constructs new languages for our experience of the world. This book has focused instead on bioethicists vying to redescribe the world: not to capture its essence, but to construct a world for their theories to thrive in—and a world where alternative theories will either struggle or starve.

In order to characterize this process, I wish to borrow another concept from Rorty, a concept that he himself borrows from literary critic Harold Bloom: the notion of a "strong poet." While Rorty leaves behind Bloom's complex Freudian-Kabbalistic-Gnostic-influenced ratios, he engages Bloom's insight that new poets must, in some manner, misread prior poets in order to create a space for themselves. Bloom's version of intertextuality imputes an emotional anxiety to creators when they are faced with prior texts;[31] strong poets must rewrite their predecessors in a manner that creates space for their own writing. For Rorty, within the context of philosophy, strong poets are those philosophers who are able to provide a better vocabulary to respond to our world—or who effectively "redescribe lots and lots of things in new ways," as Rorty puts it.[32]

To embrace how a bioethicist sees the world is, in turn, to adopt their particular moral perspective. In this book, I have tried to show how, through history, metaphors, anecdotes, dissociations, and summaries, bioethicists accomplish descriptions of the world that best suit their theory. In classic philosophical terms, David Hume famously asserted that one cannot get an "ought" from an "is"; a description of the world holds no indication of any particular moral leaning, no embedded sign of how such a world *should* be. In bioethics, while the ought comes after the is, the ought actually directs the description of is—and it is this description, I argue, that is the most powerful rhetorical technique available to the bioethicist. The strong bioethicist poet is able to redescribe the world so that their theory seems natural and self-evident.

This book has analyzed the field's most influential and widely cited texts. This has been on purpose. One reason is to show that redescription and its rhetorical components are part of mainstream bioethics discourse (and using the most familiar texts also helps to make the argument more accessible). The more important reason for my selection is to demonstrate that these bioethicists have also been, in the Rortian sense, particularly strong poets.

As mentioned in the introduction to this book, bioethicists must create a world in their text to show how their theories resolve problems in the real world. Engelhardt constructs a chaotic fallen Western world that requires a minimal morality to permit peaceful cohabitation among conflicting worldviews. Emanuel places us in a New England town hall meeting, where a communal agreement on values can be reached. Singer throws us into a world where we witness animals' indiscriminate suffering. Veatch's is a pluralistic global world so lacking any center that it requires us to start over with a new contractual foundation. Elliott shows us a world saturated with corruption by capitalism. Pierce and Jameton describe a world in which there seems no escape from environmental devastation, even in the health-care sector. And the world in which all spheres of life are sites of women's oppression, as described by Sherwin, leads readers to understand that the real fight in bioethics is over gender equity.

Aligning the word bioethicist with poet may bring to mind Plato's famous exiling of poets from *The Republic*. In her essay "Literature, Philosophy, and Medical Ethics: Let the Dialogue Go On," Anne Hunsaker Hawkins mentions this "long-standing quarrel" between philosophers and poets in relation to bioethics. Her essay is a response to Dan Clouser's criticism of a series of essays published in the journal *Medicine and Philosophy*. Hawkins had co-edited a special issue with Clouser on literature and bioethics, but Clouser seemed displeased with the manner in which bioethics issues were analyzed by the various contributors.[33] Hawkins noted the parallel between Clouser's attack and that of Plato.

> Plato resolved the quarrel by banishing literature from his ideal state, a solution that enshrined logical argumentation as the only method appropriate to the discussion of moral issues. Philosophers like Dan Clouser might prefer that the poets stay banished from the field of ethical inquiry. "We'll let you back in," he claims, "if you'll only accept our assumptions and use our methodologies." But this is to deny the unique ways in which literature and literary ways of knowing can contribute to ethics.[34]

Clouser, a philosopher, seemed to expect these essays to position literature as a helpful addition to the work of philosophers—and was surprised when the essays advanced literature as an *alternative* to philosophical bioethics, not its helpmate. Clouser essentially says that these essays have nothing substantive to add to the conversation concerning method in bioethics because, well, they do not make arguments the way philosophers do. But why, a reader might ask, are these authors (or any authors) required to draw upon the method of philosophy in discussing bioethics? Clouser makes a historical claim that ethics is philosophy; and while he is careful to point out that in its original form bioethics (at least in the United States) did not feature many philosophers, he argues that those who did bioethics—whether theologians, lawyers, physicians, and so on—still drew upon the methods originated and developed by philosophers. There are some serious flaws in this historical account. For one, early textbooks in bioethics did draw at first on deontological and utilitarian methods, but they were soon joined by a number of methods that did not have their roots in philosophy, including care ethics (moral psychology), casuistry (Catholic theology), hermeneutics (literary criticism), and communitarianism (political philosophy). In her response, Hawkins makes an interesting rhetorical move, one very much in keeping with the argument of this book: she redescribes the history of ethics in the Western tradition. Contra Clouser's history, Hawkins claims that literature, in fact, has been the "primary source of ethical wisdom throughout the history of Western civilization."[35] She points out how the ethical teaching in the Judeo-Christian tradition is rooted in stories and observes how, even in the classical Greek world from which Clouser argues, it was narratives that initiated the ongoing conversation on morality in the West. After all, that Greek world derived as much, if not more, from the work of Aeschylus, Sophocles, and Euripides than from Plato and Aristotle: "Literature holds a prior claim, a claim that is equal if not stronger."[36] In this redescription of the history of ethics, Hawkins, I believe, wins the argument—ironically, by being the stronger poet.

Of course, as has often been noted, Plato's work is filled with literary devices and rhetorical flourishes.[37] As Hawkins notes in her response to Clouser, Plato was himself "an aspiring if unsuccessful author of dramatic poetry in his youth,"[38] and his poetic abilities can be found throughout his dialogues. As discussed in the chapter on anagnorisis, Plato's famous allegory of the cave portrays human prisoners as being deceived into thinking that the shadows they watch dancing across the cave's wall are, in fact, reality. It is only when their shackles are cast off and they escape, passing by the shadowmakers as they reach the true light of the sun outside the cave, that they are able to experience the truth. It seems clear that the ones casting the shadows in front of the prisoners are the poets that Plato wishes fervently to throw out of his Republic. But as is easy to see, Plato is himself casting a shadow on the wall about shadows being cast on the wall.

When I was a child, my family traveled for weeks each year through different parts of the world. At the time, such travel was unusual. One year, I was taken to spend some time in Bali, and while there, my father purchased a shadow puppet for me, which I have sadly lost since. While Java shares with Bali the same art of shadow puppetry, there is a tradition in the Javanese version by which the audience can watch the puppet show from either side of the curtain. They can sit and simply watch the story unfold, or they can sit behind the screen with the puppeteer, watching not only the story but also how the illusion is created. This book has attempted to provide some methods by which we can view bioethics from the other side of the screen, to see how an argument is made persuasive by attending to the rhetorical mechanics that are manipulated to construct a world. In Plato's cave analogy, there was the light created by those showing the images on the wall, and there was the true light that existed outside of the cave, the world that can only be revealed through philosophy. The possibility of that truth is outside the scope of this book. Instead, it has had a far more modest objective: to, as in a Javanese shadow play, go behind the people projecting the images on the cave wall and see the mechanics by which they achieve their effects.

NOTES

1. Judith Jarvis Thomson, "A Defense of Abortion," *Philosophy and Public Affairs* 1, no. 1 (1971): 49.

2. John T. Wilcox, "Nature as Demonic in Thomson's Defense of Abortion," in *The Ethics of Abortion: Pro-Life vs. Pro-Choice*, ed. Robert M. Baird and Stuart E. Rosenbaum (Buffalo, NY: Prometheus Books, 1993), 214.

3. Wilcox, "Nature as Demonic in Thomson's Defense of Abortion," 214.

4. Katie Watson states that Thomson "posits a parallel universe." Katie Watson, *Scarlet A: The Ethics, Law and Politics of Ordinary Abortion* (New York: Oxford University Press, 2018), 112.

5. Jonathan D. Culler, *On Deconstruction: Theory and Criticism After Structuralism* (Ithaca, NY: Cornell University Press, 1983), 123–124.

6. Sidney Callahan, "Abortion and the Sexual Agenda," in *The Ethics of Abortion: Pro-Life vs. Pro-Choice*, ed. Robert M. Baird and Stuart E. Rosenbaum (Buffalo, NY: Prometheus Books, 1993), 112.

7. Callahan, "Abortion and the Sexual Agenda," 116.

8. Gregg Easterbrook, "Abortion and Brain Waves," *The New Republic*, January 31, 2000, 21.

9. Easterbrook, "Abortion and Brain Waves," 25.

10. Charles A. Gardner, "Is an Embryo a Person," *Nation* 249, no. 16 (1989): 557.

11. Easterbrook, "Abortion and Brain Waves," 25.

12. Watson, *Scarlet A: The Ethics, Law and Politics of Ordinary Abortion*, 20.

13. It needs to be noted that Watson wrote this work prior to the overturning of *Roe v. Wade* in the United States.

14. Watson, *Scarlet A: The Ethics, Law and Politics of Ordinary Abortion*, 21.

15. Watson, *Scarlet A: The Ethics, Law and Politics of Ordinary Abortion*, 21.

16. Philip J. Ivanhoe, "A Confucian Perspective on Abortion," *Dao* 9, no. 1 (2010): 42.

17. David A. Grimes and Linda G. Brandon, *Every Third Woman in America: How Legal Abortion Transformed Our Nation* (Carolina Beach, NC: Daymark Publishing, 2014).

18. Gary Leber, "We Must Rescue Them," *The Hastings Center Report* 19, no. 6 (1989): 27.

19. Don Marquis, "Why Abortion is Immoral," in *Applied Ethics, ed. Larry May and Jill B. Delston* (New York: Routledge, 2017), 367–373.

20. Albert R. Jonsen and Stephen Edelston Toulmin, *The Abuse of Casuistry: A History of Moral Reasoning* (Berkeley, CA: University of California Press, 1988).

21. Louis A. Montrose, "Professing the Renaissance: The Poetics and Politics of Culture," in *The New Historicism*, ed. H. Aram Vesser (New York: Routledge, 2013), 23.

22. Richard M. Zaner, *Ethics and the Clinical Encounter* (Englewood, NJ: Prentice Hall College Div, 1988), 27.

23. Alise L. Carse, "The "Voice of Care': Implications for Bioethical Education," *Journal of Medicine & Philosophy* 16, no. 1 (1991): 17.

24. Joseph J. Fins and Frank G. Miller, "Clinical Pragmatism, Ethics Consultation, and the Elderly Patient," *Clinics in Geriatric Medicine* 16, no. 1 (February 2000): 72.

25. D. Micah Hester, *Community as Healing: Pragmatist Ethics in Medical Encounters* (Lanham, MD: Rowman & Littlefield, 2001), 27.

26. Howard Brody, *Stories of Sickness*, 2nd ed. (Oxford: Oxford University Press, 2003), 218.

27. Larry R. Churchill, "Narrative Ethics, Gene Stories, and the Hermeneutics of Consent Forms," in *Stories Matter* (New York: Routledge, 2004), 189.

28. Tom L. Beauchamp and James F. Childress, *Principles of Biomedical Ethics*, 5th ed. (New York: Oxford University Press, 2001), 15.

29. Susan Sherwin, *No Longer Patient: Feminist Ethics and Health Care* (Philadelphia, PA: Temple University Press, 1992), 79–80.

30. Margaret Urban Walker, "Introduction: Groningen Naturalism in Bioethics," in *Naturalized Bioethics: Toward Responsible Knowing and Practice*, ed. Hilde Lindemann, Marian Verkerk, and Margaret Urban Walker (Cambridge: Cambridge University Press, 2008), 10.

31. See Harold Bloom, *The Anxiety of Influence: A Theory of Poetry*, 2nd ed. (New York: Oxford University Press, 1997).

32. Richard Rorty, *Contingency, Irony, and Solidarity* (Cambridge; New York: Cambridge University Press, 1989), 9.

33. It seems necessary to mention that the author of this monograph was one of the contributors to this special issue that Clouser found wanting.

34. Anne Hunsaker Hawkins, "Literature, Philosophy, and Medical Ethics: Let the Dialogue Go On," *Journal of Medicine and Philosophy* 21, no. 3 (1996): 341.

35. Hawkins, "Literature, Philosophy, and Medical Ethics: Let the Dialogue Go On," 341–342.

36. Hawkins, "Literature, Philosophy, and Medical Ethics: Let the Dialogue Go On," 342.

37. In *Genres in Dialogue*, Andrew Wilson Nightingale argues that Plato creatively and explicitly engages other literary genres in order to define, through its intertextual construction, philosophy. Andrea Wilson Nightingale, *Genres in Dialogue: Plato and the Construct of Philosophy* (Cambridge; New York: Cambridge University Press, 1995).

38. Hawkins, "Literature, Philosophy, and Medical Ethics: Let the Dialogue Go On," 341.

Bibliography

Abbott, H. Porter. *The Cambridge Introduction to Narrative.* Cambridge; New York: Cambridge University Press, 2002.

Althouse, Matthew T., and Floyd D. Anderson. "“Trouble with a Capital T”: Jerome S Bruner's Reenvisioning of Kenneth Burke's Dramatistic Pentad." *K.B. Journal* 11, no. 2 (Spring 2016). Accessed November 14, 2022. http://www.kbjournal.org/althouse-anderson.

Amdur, Robert J., and Elizabeth A. Bankert. *Institutional Review Board: Member Handbook.* Burlington, VT: Jones & Bartlett Learning, 2022.

Amsterdam, Anthony G., and Jerome S. Bruner. *Minding the Law.* Cambridge, MA: Harvard University Press, 2000.

Anderson, Floyd D. "Five Fingers or Six? Pentad or Hexad?" *KB Journal* 6, no. 2. (2010): NP. https://kbjournal.org/anderson.

Andre, Judith. *Bioethics as Practice.* Chapel Hill, NC: University of North Carolina Press, 2002.

Annas, George J. "Scientific Discoveries and Cloning: Challenges for Public Policy." In *Flesh of My Flesh: The Ethics of Cloning Humans*, edited by Gregory E. Pence, 77–84. Lanham, MD: Rowman & Littlefield, 1998.

Aristotle. *The Complete Works of Aristotle: The Revised Oxford Translation. Vol. 2.* Edited by Jonathan Barnes. Princeton, NJ: Princeton University Press, 1984.

Arras, John D. "Getting Down to Cases: The Revival of Casuistry in Bioethics." *Journal of Medicine and Philosophy* 16, no. 1 (February 1991): 29–51.

———. "The Hedgehog and the Borg: Common Morality in Bioethics." *Theoretical Medicine and Bioethics* 30 (2009): 11–30.

———. "Nice Story, but So What? Narrative and Justification in Ethics." In *Stories and Their Limits: Narrative Approaches to Bioethics*, edited by Hilde Lindemann Nelson, 65–88. New York: Routleldge, 2014.

Baker, Robert. *The Structure of Moral Revolutions: Studies of Changes in the Morality of Abortion, Death, and the Bioethics Revolution.* Cambridge, MA: The MIT Press, 2019.

Barnard, David. "Reflections of a Reluctant Clinical Ethicist: Ethics Consultation and the Collapse of Critical Distance." *Theoretical Medicine* 13 (1992): 15–22.

Barthes, Roland. "From Work to Text." Translated by Stephen Heath. In *The Pleasure of the Text*, 155–164. New York: Hill and Wang, 1975.

Battin, Margaret Pabst. *The Death Debate: Ethical Issues in Suicide.* Upper Saddle River, NJ: Prentice Hall, 1996.

Beauchamp, Tom L. "A Defense of the Common Morality." *Kennedy Institute of Ethics Journal* 13, no. 3 (2003): 259–274.

———. "The Origins and Evolution of the Belmont Report." In *Belmont Revisited*, edited by James F. Childress, Eric M. Meslin and Harold T. Shapiro, 12–25. Washington, DC: Georgetown University Press, 2005.

Beauchamp, Tom L., and James F. Childress. *Principles of Biomedical Ethics.* New York: Oxford University Press, 2019.

———. *Principles of Biomedical Ethics.* 4th ed. New York: Oxford University Press, 1994.

———. *Principles of Biomedical Ethics.* 5th ed. New York: Oxford University Press, 2001.

Beecher, Henry K. "After the Definition of Irreversible Coma." *The New England Journal of Medicine* 281 (1969): 1070–1071.

———. "A Definition of Irreversible Coma: Report of the Ad Hoc Committee of the Harvard Medical School to Examine the Definition of Brain Death." *Journal of the American Medical Association* 205, no. 6 (1968): 337–340.

Bernat, James L., Charles M. Culver, and Bernard Gert. "On the Definition and Criterion of Death." *Annals of Internal Medicine* 94, no. 3 (1981): 389–394.

Berry, Franklin M. "An Introduction to Stephen C. Pepper's Philosophical System Via World Hypotheses: A Study in Evidence." *Bulletin of the Psychonomic Society* 22, no. 5 (1984): 446–448.

Bilsky, Manuel, McCrea Hazlett, Robert E. Streeter, and Richard M. Weaver. "Looking for an Argument." *College English* 14 (1953): 210–216.

Bliese, John R. E. "Richard Weaver's Axiology of Argument." *Southern Speech Communication Journal* 44, no. 3 (1979): 275–288.

Bloom, Harold. *The Anxiety of Influence: A Theory of Poetry.* 2nd ed. New York: Oxford University Press, 1997.

Borges, Jorge Louis. "Kafka and His Precursors." In *Labyrinths*, 199–201. New York: New Directions, 1964.

Brock, Dan W. "Active Voluntary Euthanasia." *Hastings Center Report* 22, no. 2 (March–April 1992): 10–22.

Brody, Baruch A. *Life and Death Decision Making.* Oxford: Oxford University Press, 1988.

Brody, Howard. *Stories of Sickness.* 2nd ed. Oxford: Oxford University Press, 2003.

Brummett, Barry. "Burke's Representative Anecdote as a Method in Media Criticism." *Critical Studies in Mass Communication* 1, no. 2 (2009): 161–176.

———. "A Pentadic Analysis of Ideologies in Two Gay Rights Controversies." *Central States Speech Journal* 30, no. 3 (1979): 250–261.

Burke, Kenneth. *A Grammar of Motives*. Berkeley, CA: University of California Press, 1969.

———. *Permanence and Change: An Anatomy of Purpose*. 3rd ed. Berkeley, CA: University of California Press, 1984.

———. "Questions and Answers About the Pentad." *College Composition and Communication* 29, no. 4 (1978): 330–335.

Cahill, Lisa Sowle. "Abortion and Argument by Analogy." *Horizons* 9, no. 2 (1982): 271–287.

Callahan, Sidney. "Abortion and the Sexual Agenda." In *The Ethics of Abortion: Pro-Life Vs. Pro-Choice*, edited by Robert M. Baird and Stuart E. Rosenbaum, 111–121. Buffalo, NY: Prometheus Books, 1993.

Caplan, Arthur L. "Can Applied Ethics Be Effective in Health Care and Should It Strive to Be?" *Ethics* 93, no. 2 (1983): 311–319.

———."Ethical Engineers Need Not Apply: The State of Applied Ethics Today." *Science, Technology & Human Values* 5, no. 4 (1980): 24–32.

Carlin, David R. "Rights, Animal and Human." *First Things: A Monthly Journal of Religion and Public Life* 105 (2000): 16–17.

Carroll, Lewis. *Sylvie and Bruno Concluded*. London: Macmillan, 1895.

Carse, Alise L. "The 'Voice of Care': Implications for Bioethical Education." *Journal of Medicine & Philosophy* 16, no. 1 (1991): 5–28.

Cash, John. "The Case Study as Representative Anecdote." In *Case Studies and the Dissemination of Knowledge*, edited by Joy Damousi, Birgit Lang, and Katie Sutton, 31–48. New York: Routledge, 2015.

Cave, Terence. *Recognitions: A Study in Poetics*. Oxford: Clarendon Press, 1988.

Chambers, Tod. *The Fiction of Bioethics*. New York: Routledge, 1999.

———. "Framing Our Mistakes." In *Margin of Error: The Necessity, Inevitability, and Ethics of Mistakes in Medicine and Bioethics Consultation*, edited by Susan Rubin and Laurie Zoloth, 13–24. Frederick, MD: University Publishing Group, 2000.

The Chicago Manual of Style. Chicago, IL: University of Chicago Press, 2017.

Childress, James F. *Practical Reasoning in Bioethics*. Medical Ethics Series. Bloomington, IN: Indiana University Press, 1997.

———. "Principles-Oriented Bioethics: An Analysis and Assessment from Within." In *A Matter of Principles?: Ferment in U.S. Bioethics*, edited by Edwin R. DuBose, Ronald P. Hamel, and Laurence J. O'Connell, 72–98. Valley Forge, PA: Trinity Press International, 1994.

Churchill, Larry R. "The Ethicist in Professional Education." *Hastings Center Report* 8 (1978): 13–15.

———. "Narrative Ethics, Gene Stories, and the Hermeneutics of Consent Forms." In *Stories Matter*, edited by Rita Charon and Martha Montello, 201–213. London: Routledge, 2004.

Clouser, K. Danner. "Philosophy, Literature, and Ethics: Let the Engagement Begin." *The Journal of Medicine and Philosophy* 21, no. 3 (1996): 321–340.

Clouser, K. Danner, and Bernard Gert. "A Critique of Principlism." *The Journal of Medicine and Philosophy* 15, no. 2 (1990): 219–236.

Clouser, K. Danner, and Anne Hunsaker Hawkins. "Literature and Medical Ethics." *The Journal of Medicine and Philosophy* 21, no. 3 (1996): 237–241.

Cohen, Carl. "In Defense of the Use of Animals." In *The Animal Rights Debate*, edited by Carl Cohen and Tom Regan, 3–123. Lanham, MD: Rowman & Littlefield, 2006.

Crouch, Robert. "Let the Deaf Be Deaf: Reconsidering the Use of Cochlear Implants in Prelingually Deaf Children." *Hastings Center Report* 27, no. 4 (1997): 14–21.

Culler, Jonathan D. *On Deconstruction: Theory and Criticism after Structuralism.* Ithaca, NY: Cornell University Press, 1983.

Culver, Charles M., and Bernard Gert. *Philosophy in Medicine: Conceptual and Ethical Issues in Medicine and Psychiatry.* New York: Oxford University Press, 1982.

Daniels, Norman. *Just Health Care.* Studies in Philosophy and Health Policy. Cambridge; New York: Cambridge University Press, 1985.

Danto, Arthur C. *Narration and Knowledge.* New York: Columbia University Press, 2007.

Davis, Richard B. "The Principlism Debate: A Critical Overview." *The Journal of Medicine and Philosophy* 20, no. 1 (1995): 85–105.

Drane, James F. "Character and the Moral Life: A Virtue Approach to Biomedical Ethics." Chap. 12 In *A Matter of Principles?: Ferment in U.S. Bioethics*, edited by E. R. DuBose, R. P. Hamel, and L. J. O'Connel, 284–309. Valley Forge, PA: Trinity, 1994.

DuBose, Edwin R., Ronald P. Hamel, and Laurence J. O'Connell, eds. "Introduction." In *A Matter of Principles?: Ferment in U.S. Bioethics*, edited by E. R. DuBose, R. P. Hamel, and L. J. O'Connel, 1–17. Valley Forge, PA: Trinity, 1994.

Durkheim, Emile. *On Suicide.* Translated by Robin Buss. London: Penguin, 2006.

Easterbrook, Gregg. "Abortion and Brain Waves." *The New Republic*, January 31, 2000, 21–25.

Eemeren, Frans H. van, Bart Garssen, Erik C. W. Krabbe, A. Francisca Snoeck Henkemans, Bart Verheij, and Jean H. M. Wagemans. *Handbook of Argumentation Theory: A Critical Survey of Classical Backgrounds and Modern Studies.* Dordrecht: Springer, 1987.

Elliott, Carl. *White Coat, Black Hat: Adventures on the Dark Side of Medicine.* Boston, MA: Beacon Press, 2010.

Emanuel, Ezekiel J. *The Ends of Human Life: Medical Ethics in a Liberal Polity.* Cambridge, MA: Harvard University Press, 1991.

Engelhardt, H. Tristram. *The Foundations of Bioethics.* 2nd ed. New York: Oxford University Press, 1996.

———. *The Foundations of Christian Bioethics.* Lisse: Swets & Zeitlinger, 2000.

Engelhardt Jr, H. Tristram. "The Search for a Universal System of Ethics: Post-Modern Disappointments and Contemporary Possibilities." In *Ethical Problems in Dialysis and Transplantation*, edited by Carl M. Kjellstrand and John B. Dossetor, 3–19. Dordrecht: Springer, 1992.

Evans, John Hyde. *The History and Future of Bioethics: A Sociological View.* New York: Oxford University Press, 2012.

———. "A Sociological Account of the Growth of Principlism." *Hastings Center Report* 30, no. 5 (September–October 2000): 31–38.

Fins, Joseph J., and Frank G. Miller. "Clinical Pragmatism, Ethics Consultation, and the Elderly Patient." *Clinics in Geriatric Medicine* 16, no. 1 (February 2000): 71–81.

Fletcher, Joseph F. *Humanhood: Essays in Biomedical Ethics.* Buffalo, NY: Prometheus Books, 1979.

———. *Morals and Medicine.* Boston, MA: Beacon Press, 1960.

Foss, Sonja K. "Abandonment of Genus: The Evolution of Political Rhetoric." *Communication Studies* 33, no. 2 (1982): 367–378.

———. *Rhetorical Criticism: Exploration and Practice.* 5th ed. Long Grove, IL: Waveland Press, 2008.

Foss, Sonja K., Karen A. Foss, and Robert Trapp. *Contemporary Perspectives on Rhetoric.* 3rd ed. Prospect Heights, IL: Waveland Press, 2002.

Fowles, John. *The French Lieutenant's Woman.* Boston, MA: Little, Brown & Company, 1969.

Fox, Renee. "The Evolution of American Bioethics: A Sociological Perspective." In *Social Science Perspectives on Medical Ethics*, edited by George Weisz, 201–217. Dordrecht; Boston, MA: Kluwer Academic Publishers, 1990.

Fox, Renée C., and Judith P. Swazey. "Medical Morality Is Not Bioethics: Medical Ethics in China and the United States." *Perspectives in Biology and Medicine* 27 (1984): 336–360.

Fox, Renée C., Judith P. Swazey, and Judith C. Watkins. *Observing Bioethics.* Oxford: Oxford University Press, 2008.

Frank, Arthur W. *The Wounded Storyteller: Body, Illness, and Ethics.* Chicago, IL: University of Chicago Press, 1995.

Frye, Northrop. *Anatomy of Criticism: Four Essays.* Princeton, NJ: Princeton University Press, 1957.

Gardner, Charles A. "Is an Embryo a Person." *Nation* 249, no. 16 (1989): 557–559.

Gaylin, Willard, Leon R. Kass, Edmund D. Pellegrino, and Mark Siegler. "Doctors Must Not Kill'." *Journal of the American Medical Association* 259, no. 14 (1988): 2139–2140.

Geertz, Clifford. *Works and Lives: The Anthropologist as Author.* Stanford, CA: Stanford University Press, 1988.

Genette, Gérard. *Palimpsests: Literature in the Second Degree.* Translated by Channa Newman and Claude Doubinsky. Lincoln, NE: University of Nebraska Press, 1997.

Gert, Bernard, and Bernard Gert. *Morality: A New Justification of the Moral Rules.* New York: Oxford University Press, 1988.

Gert, Bernard, Charles M. Culver, and K. Danner Clouser. *Bioethics: A Return to Fundamentals.* New York: Oxford University Press, 1997.

———. *Bioethics: A Systematic Approach.* 2nd ed. New York: Oxford University Press, 2006.

Gilles, Roger. "Richard Weaver Revisited: Rhetoric Left, Right, and Middle." *Rhetoric Review* 15, no. 1 (1996): 128–141.

Gillett, Grant. *Bioethics in the Clinic: Hippocratic Reflections*. Baltimore, MD: Johns Hopkins University Press, 2004.

Gilligan, Carol. *In a Different Voice: Psychological Theory and Women's Development*. Acls Humanities E-Book. 38th print ed. Cambridge, MA: Harvard University Press, 2003.

Graber, Glenn. "The Rationality of Suicide." In *Suicide and Euthanasia: The Rights of Personhood*, edited by Albin Eser and Samuel E. Wallace, 51–65. Knoxville, TN: University of Tennesse Press, 1981.

Grimes, David A., and Linda G. Brandon. *Every Third Woman in America: How Legal Abortion Transformed Our Nation*. Carolina Beach: Daymark Publishing, 2014.

Grodin, Michael A., and Harlan L. Lane. "Ethical Issues in Cochlear Implant Surgery: An Exploration into Disease, Disability, and the Best Interests of the Child." *Kennedy Institute of Ethics Journal* 7, no. 3 (1997): 231–251.

Gross, Alan G., and Ray D. Dearin. *Chaim Perelman*. Albany, NY: State University of New York Press, 2003.

Gusfield, Joseph R. *The Culture of Public Problems: Drinking-Driving and the Symbolic Order*. Chicago, IL: University of Chicago Press, 1981.

———. "Introduction." In *On Symbols and Society*, edited by Joseph R. Gusfield, 1–49. Chicago, IL: University of Chicago Press, 1989.

Halpern, Jodi. *From Detached Concern to Empathy: Humanizing Medical Practice*. Oxford: Oxford University Press, 2001.

Hawkins, Anne Hunsaker. "Literature, Philosophy, and Medical Ethics: Let the Dialogue Go On." *Journal of Medicine and Philosophy* 21, no. 3 (1996): 341–354.

Hayes, Steven C., Linda J. Hayes, and Hayne W. Reese. "Finding the Philosophical Core: A Review of Stephen C. Pepper's World Hypotheses: A Study in Evidence." *Journal of the Experimental Analysis of Behavior* 50, no. 1 (1988): 97.

Hester, D. Micah. *Community as Healing: Pragmatist Ethics in Medical Encounters*. Lanham, MD: Rowman & Littlefield, 2001.

Hofmann, B., J. H. Solbakk, and S. Holm. "Teaching Old Dogs New Tricks: The Role of Analogies in Bioethical Analysis and Argumentation Concerning New Technologies." *Theorectical Medicine and Bioethics* 27, no. 5 (2006): 397–413.

Hunter, Kathryn Montgomery. "Narrative." In *Encyclopedia of Bioethics*, edited by Warrant T. Reich, 1791–1794. New York: Simon & Schuster, 1995.

Huxtable, Richard, and Jonathan Ives. "License to Kill: A New Model for Excusing Medically Assisted Dying?" In *New Directions in the Ethics of Assisted Suicide and Euthanasia*, edited by Michael Cholbi and Jukka Varelius, 149–168. Cham: Springer, 2015.

Ilea, Ramona. "Singer, Wittgenstein, and Morally Motivating Examples." *Between the Species* 22, no. 1 (2017): 1.

Ivanhoe, Philip J. "A Confucian Perspective on Abortion." *Dao* 9, no. 1 (2010): 37–51.

Jaggar, Alison M. "Abortion and a Woman's Right to Decide." In *Living with Contradictions*, edited by Alison M. Jaggar, 281–287. Boulder, CO: Westview Press, 1994.

———. "Regendering the Us Abortion Debate." *Journal of social philosophy* 28, no. 1 (1997): 127–140.

Jameston, Andrew, and Albert R. Jonsen. "America, Bioethics In." In *Bioethics*, edited by Bruce Jennings, 184–202. Farmington Hills, MI: Macmillan Reference, Gale, Cengage Learning, 2014.

Johannesen, Richard L. "Richard M. Weaver on Standards for Ethical Rhetoric." *Communication Studies* 29, no. 2 (1978): 127–137.

———. "Richard Weaver's View of Rhetoric and Criticism." *Southern Journal of Communication* 32, no. 2 (1966): 133–145.

Johannesen, Richard L., Rennard Strickland, and Ralph T. Eubanks. "Richard M. Weaver on the Nature of Rhetoric: An Interpretation." In *Language Is Sermonic: Richard M. Weaver on the Nature of Rhetoric*, edited by Richard L. Johannesen, Rennard Strickland, and Ralph T. Eubanks, 7–30. Baton Rouge, FL: Louisiana State University Press, 1985.

Jonsen, Albert R. "The Birth of Bioethics." *Hastings Center Report* 23, no. 6 (November–December 1993): S1–S4.

———. *The Birth of Bioethics.* New York: Oxford University Press, 1998.

———. "Casuistry: An Alternative or Complement to Principles?" *Kennedy Institute of Ethics Journal* 5, no. 3 (1995): 237–251.

———. "Casuistry and Clinical Ethics." *Theoretical Medicine* 7 (1986): 65–74.

———. "Casuistry as Methodology in Clinical Ethics." *Theoretical Medicine* 12, no. 4 (1991): 295–307.

———. *The New Medicine and the Old Ethics.* Cambridge, MA: Harvard University Press, 1990.

———. *The New Medicine and the Old Ethics.* Cambridge, MA: Harvard University Press, 1992.

Jonsen, Albert R., Mark Siegler, and William J. Winslade. *Clinical Ethics: A Practical Approach to Ethical Decisions in Clinical Medicine.* 3rd ed. New York: McGraw-Hill Health Professions Division, 1992.

Jonsen, Albert R., and Stephen Edelston Toulmin. *The Abuse of Casuistry: A History of Moral Reasoning.* Berkeley, CA: University of California Press, 1988.

Kaebnick, Gregory E. *Humans in Nature: The World as We Find It and the World as We Create It.* New York: Oxford University Press, 2014.

Kass, Leon R. "Implications of Prenatal Diagnosis for the Human Right to Life." In *Biomedical Ethics and the Law*, edited by James M. Humber and Robert F. Almeder, 335–349. Boston, MA: Springer, 1979.

———. *Toward a More Natural Science: Biology and Human Affairs.* New York: Free Press, 1985.

———. "The Wisdom of Repugnance: Why We Should Ban the Cloning of Humans." *New Republic* 216, no. 22 (1997): 17–26.

Kaveney, Roz. *From Alien to the Matrix: Reading Science Fiction Film.* London: I.B. Tauris, 2005.

Kermode, Frank. *The Sense of an Ending: Studies in the Theory of Fiction.* New York: Oxford University Press, 1967.

Kierkegaard, Søren. *Parables of Kierkegaard.* Edited by Thomas C. Oden. Princeton, NJ: Princeton University Press, 1978.

Kleinman, Arthur. *Writing at the Margin: Discourse between Anthropology and Medicine.* Berkeley, CA: University of California Press, 1995.

Klugman, Craig M. "Blood Donation and Its Metaphors." *The American Journal of Bioethics* 10, no. 2 (2010): 46–47.

Koch, Tom. "The Hippocratic Thorn in Bioethics' Hide: Cults, Sects, and Strangeness." *Journal of Medicine and Philosophy* 39, no. 1 (February 2014): 75–88.

Kripke, Saul A. *Naming and Necessity.* Cambridge, MA: Harvard University Press, 1980.

Kuczewski, Mark. "Casuistry and Principlism: The Convergence of Method in Biomedical Ethics." *Theoretical Medicine and Bioethics* 19, no. 6 (1998): 509–524.

Landau, Misia. "Human Evolution as Narrative." In *Memory, Identity, Community: The Idea of Narrative in the Human Sciences*, edited by Lewis P. Hinchman and Sandra K. Hinchman, 104–118. New Haven, CT: Yale University Press, 1997.

Lantos, John D. *Do We Still Need Doctors?* New York: Routledge, 1997.

Leber, Gary. "We Must Rescue Them." *The Hastings Center Report* 19, no. 6 (1989): 26–27.

Leder, Drew. *The Distressed Body: Rethinking Illness, Imprisonment, and Healing.* Chicago, IL: University of Chicago Press, 2016.

———. "Toward a Hermeneutical Bioethics." Chap. 10 In *A Matter of Principles?: Ferment in U.S. Bioethics*, edited by E. R. DuBose, R. P. Hamel, and L. J. O'Connel, 240–259. Valley Forg, PA: Trinity, 1994.

Lindemann Nelson, Hilde. *Damaged Identities, Narrative Repair.* Ithaca, NY: Cornell University Press, 2001.

Ling, David A. "A Pentadic Analysis of Senator Edward Kennedy's Address to the People of Massachusetts, July 25, 1969." *Communication Studies* 21, no. 2 (1970): 81–86.

Lodge, David. *The Art of Fiction: Illustrated from Classic and Modern Texts.* New York: Viking, 1993.

———. *Working with Structuralism: Essays and Reviews on Nineteenth and Twentieth-Century Literature.* London: Routledge & Kegan Paul, 1981.

MacDonald, Chris. "Will the "Secular Priests" of Bioethics Work among the Sinners?" *American Journal of Bioethics* 3, no. 2 (2003): 36–39.

Macklin, Ruth. *Mortal Choices: Bioethics in Today's World.* New York: Pantheon Books, 1987.

Madsen, Arnie. "Burke's Representative Anecdote as a Critical Method." In *Extensions of the Burkean System*, edited by James W. Cheseboro, 208–229. Tuscaloosa, AL: University of Alabama Press, 1993.

Manson, Neil C., and Onora O'Neill. *Rethinking Informed Consent in Bioethics.* Cambridge: Cambridge University Press, 2007.

Marquis, Don. "Why Abortion Is Immoral." In *Applied Ethics*, edited by Larry May and Jill B. Delston, 367–373. New York: Routledge, 2017.

May, Alexis M., and E. David Klonsky. "What Distinguishes Suicide Attempters from Suicide Ideators? A Meta-Analysis of Potential Factors." *Clinical Psychology: Science and Practice* 23, no. 1 (2016): 5.

May, William F. "Code, Covenant, Contract, or Philanthropy." *Hastings Center Report* 5 (December 1975): 29–38.

———. *The Physician's Covenant: Images of the Healer in Medical Ethics.* 2nd ed. Lexington, KY: Westminster John Knox Press, 2000.

McCloskey, Donald. *The Rhetoric of Economics.* Madison, WI: University of Wisconsin Press, 1985.

Mink, Louis. "Narrative Form as a Cognitive Instrument." In *The Writing of History: Literary Form and Historical Understanding*, edited by Robert H. Canary and Henry Kozicki, 140. Madison, WI: University of Wisconsin Press, 1978.

Montello, Martha. "Narrative Competence." In *Stories and Their Limits: Narrative Approaches to Bioethics*, edited by Hilde Lindemann Nelson, 185–197. London: Routledge, 1997.

Montrose, Louis A. "Professing the Renaissance: The Poetics and Politics of Culture." In *The New Historicism*, edited by H. Aram Vesser, 15–36. New York: Routledge, 2013.

Morreim, E. Haavi. *Balancing Act: The New Medical Ethics of Medicine's New Economics.* Washington, DC: Georgetown University Press, 1995.

Murray, Thomas H. "What Do We Mean by Ethics and Narrative?" In *Stories and Their Limits: Narrative Approaches to Bioethics*, edited by Hilde Lindemann Nelson, 3–17. New York: Routledge, 1997.

Nelson, Hilde Lindemann. "Four Narrative Approaches to Bioethics." In *Handbook of Bioethics*, edited by George Khushf, 163–181. New York: Kluwer Springer, 2004.

Nelson, John S., Allan Megill, and Donald N. McCloskey. "Rhetoric of Inquiry." In *The Rhetoric of the Human Sciences: Language and Argument in Scholarship and Public Affairs*, edited by John S. Nelson, Allan Megill, and Donald N. McCloskey. 3–18 Madison, WI: University of Wisconsin Press, 1987.

Nightingale, Andrea Wilson. *Genres in Dialogue: Plato and the Construct of Philosophy.* Cambridge; New York: Cambridge University Press, 1995.

Noddings, Nel. *Caring: A Feminine Approach to Ethics and Moral Education.* 2nd Rev. ed. Berkeley, CA: University of California Press, 2003.

O'Keefe, Meaghan, Sarah Perrault, Jodi Halpern, Lisa Ikemoto, and Mark Yarborough. "'Editing' Genes: A Case Study About How Language Matters in Bioethics." *The American Journal of Bioethics* 15, no. 12 (2015): 3–10.

Olson, Kathryn M. "Dissociation." In *Encyclopedia of Rhetoric and Composition: Communication from Ancient Times to the Information Age*, edited by Theresa Enos, 196–197. New York: Routledge, 2010.

Osborn, Michael. "Archetypal Metaphor in Rhetoric: The Light-Dark Family." *Quarterly Journal of Speech* 53, no. 2 (1967): 115–126.

———. "The Trajectory of My Work with Metaphor." *Southern Communication Journal* 74, no. 1 (2009): 79–87.

Parens, Erik. "Is Better Always Good?: The Enhancement Project." *Hastings Center Report* 28 (January–February 1998): S1–S15.

Pellegrino, Edmund D. "Character, Virtue and Self-Interest in the Ethics of the Professions." *The Journal of Contemporary Health Law & Policy* 5 (1989): 53.

———. "The Metamorphosis of Medical Ethics. A 30-Year Retrospective." *Journal of the American Medical Association* 269, no. 9 (Mar 3 1993): 1158–1162.

Pellegrino, Edmund D., and David C. Thomasma. *The Virtues in Medical Practice.* New York: Oxford University Press, 1993.

Pence, Gregory E. *Who's Afraid of Human Cloning?* Lanham, MD: Rowman & Littlefield, 1998.

Pepper, Stephen C. *World Hypotheses, a Study in Evidence.* Berkeley and Los Angeles, CA: University of California Press, 1942.

Perelman, Chaïm. *The Realm of Rhetoric.* Notre Dame, IN: University of Notre Dame Press, 1982.

Perelman, Chaïm, and Lucie Olbrechts-Tyteca. *The New Rhetoric: A Treatise on Argumentation.* Notre Dame, IN: University of Notre Dame Press, 1969.

Pierce, Jessica, and Andrew Jameton. *The Ethics of Environmentally Responsible Health Care.* New York: Oxford University Press, 2004.

Pincoffs, Edmund. "Quandary Ethics." *Mind* 80, no. 320 (1971): 552–571.

Pope, Thaddeus Mason. "Review of Lawrence J. Schneiderman and Nancy S. Jecker, Wrong Medicine: Doctors, Patients, and Futile Treatment." *American Journal of Bioethics* 12, no. 1 (2012): 49–51.

Rachels, James. "Active and Passive Euthanasia." *New England Journal of Medicine* 292 (9 January 1975): 78–80.

Ramsey, Paul. *Fabricated Man: The Ethics of Genetic Control.* New Haven, CT: Yale University Press, 1974.

Regan, Tom. *The Case for Animal Rights.* Updated with a new pref. ed. Berkeley, CA: University of California Press, 2004. (02) Monograph.

Rhodes, Rosamond. *The Trusted Doctor: Medical Ethics and Professionalism.* New York: Oxford University Press, 2020.

Richards, I. A. *The Philosophy of Rhetoric.* London: Oxford University Press, 1965.

Robb, J Wesley. "The Fletcher/Ramsey Debate in Bioethics and the Christian Ethical Tradition." *Religion in Life* 46, no. 1 (1977): 81–91.

Ropp, Cyd C. "Pentadic Cartography: Mapping Obstetric Medicine and Traditional Midwifery." Paper presented at the National Communication Association, New Orleans, LA, November 2002.

Rorty, Richard. *Contingency, Irony, and Solidarity.* Cambridge; New York: Cambridge University Press, 1989.

Rosenblatt, Eloise. "Book Review—Reading the Bible in the Strange World of Medicine." *Health Progress,* July–August 2005, 67–68.

Ross, Lainie Friedman. "Health Care Decisionmaking by Children Is It in Their Best Interest?" *Hastings Center Report* 27, no. 6 (1997): 41–46.

Rothman, David J. *Strangers at the Bedside: A History of How Law and Bioethics Transformed Medical Decision Making.* New York: Basic Books, 1991.

Schiappa, Edward. "Arguing About Definitions." *Argumentation* 7 (1993): 403–417.

Schneiderman, Lawrence J., and Nancy Jecker. *Wrong Medicine: Doctors, Patients, and Futile Treatment.* Baltimore, MD: Johns Hopkins University Press, 1995.

Sherwin, Susan. *No Longer Patient: Feminist Ethics and Health Care.* Philadelphia, PA: Temple University Press, 1992.

Shildrick, Margrit. *Leaky Bodies and Boundaries: Feminism, Postmodernism and (Bio)Ethics.* London: Routledge, 1997.

Siegler, Mark. "Clinical Ethics and Clinical Medicine." *Archives of Internal Medicine* 139, no. 8 (1979): 914–915.

Simons, Herbert W. *The Rhetorical Turn: Invention and Persuasion in the Conduct of Inquiry*. Chicago, IL: University of Chicago Press, 2011.

Singer, Peter. *Animal Liberation: The Definitive Classic of the Animal Movement*. Updated ed. New York: Ecco, 2009.

Sparrow, Robert. "Defending Deaf Culture: The Case of Cochlear Implants." *Journal of Political Philosophy* 13, no. 2 (2005): 135–152.

Sprinkle, Robert Hunt. "Bioethics without Analogy." In *Clinical Ethics and the Necessity of Stories: Essays in Honor of Richard M. Zaner*, edited by Osborne P. Wiggins and Annette C. Allen, 71–85. Dordrecht: Springer, 2010.

Stam, Robert. "Beyond Fidelity: The Dialogics of Adaptation." In *Film Adaptation*, edited by James Naremore, 54–76. New Brunswick, NJ: Rutgers, 2000.

Steinbock, Bonnie. "The Intentional Termination of Life." In *Killing and Letting Die*, edited by Bonnie Steinbock and Alastair Norcross. Englewood Cliffs, NJ: Prentice-Hall, 1980. 69–80.

Stevens, M. L. Tina. *Bioethics in America : Origins and Cultural Politics*. Baltimore, MD: Johns Hopkins University Press, 2000.

Thomson, Judith Jarvis. "A Defense of Abortion." *Philosophy and Public Affairs* 1, no. 1 (1971): 47.

Tomlinson, Thomas. *Methods in Medical Ethics: Critical Perspectives*. Oxford: Oxford University Press, 2012.

Tooley, Michael. "Abortion and Infanticide." *Philosophy & Public Affairs* 2 (1972): 37–65.

Toulmin, Stephen. "How Medicine Saved the Life of Ethics." *Perspectives in Biology and Medicine* 25, no. 4 (Summer 1982): 736–750.

———. *The Place of Reason in Ethics*. Cambridge: Cambridge University Press, 1970.

———. "The Tyranny of Principles." *Hastings Center Report* 11, no. 6 (1981): 31–39.

———. *The Uses of Argument*. Cambridge: Cambridge University Press, 1958.

Trotter, Griffin. *The Loyal Physician: Roycean Ethics and the Practice of Medicine*. Nashville, TN: Vanderbilt University Press, 1997.

Turner, Leigh. "Medical Facilities as Moral Worlds." *Medical humanities* 28, no. 1 (2002): 19–22.

———. "Zones of Consensus and Zones of Conflict: Questioning the "Common Morality" Presumption in Bioethics." *Kennedy Institute of Ethics Journal* 13, no. 3 (2003): 193–218.

Twine, Richard. "Constructing Critical Bioethics by Deconstructing Culture/Nature Dualism." *Medicine, Health Care and Philosophy* 8 (2005): 285–295.

Van Rees, Agnes. *Dissociation in Argumentative Discussions: A Pragma-Dialectical Perspective*. Vol. 13. Dordrecht: Springer Science & Business Media, 2008.

Veatch, Robert. *Theory of Medical Ethics*. New York: Basic Books, 1981.

Verhey, Allen. *Reading the Bible in the Strange World of Medicine*. Grand Rapids, MI: W.B. Eerdmans Pub. Co., 2003.

Veyne, Paul. *Writing History: Essay on Epistemology*. Manchester: Manchester University Press, 1984.

Walker, Margaret Urban. "Introduction: Groningen Naturalism in Bioethics." In *Naturalized Bioethics: Toward Responsible Knowing and Practice*, edited by Hilde Lindemann, Marian Verkerk, and Margaret Urban Walker, 1–20. Cambridge: Cambridge University Press, 2008.

———. *Moral Understandings: A Feminist Study in Ethics*. New York: Routledge, 1998.

Watson, Katie. *Scarlet A: The Ethics, Law and Politics of Ordinary Abortion*. New York: Oxford University Press, 2018.

Weaver, Richard M. *Composition: A Course in Writing and Rhetoric*. New York: Holt, 1957.

———. *The Ethics of Rhetoric*. Battleboro, VT: Echo Point Books & Media, 2011. 1953.

———. *Language Is Sermonic: Richard M. Weaver on the Nature of Rhetoric*. Edited by Richard L. Johannesen, Rennard Strickland, and Ralph T. Eubanks. Baton Rouge, LA: Louisiana State University Press, 1985.

———. "Two Orators." *Modern Age* 14, no. 3 (1970): 226.

White, Hayden V. *The Content of the Form: Narrative Discourse and Historical Representation*. Baltimore, MD: Johns Hopkins University Press, 1987.

———. *Metahistory: The Historical Imagination in Nineteenth-Century Europe*. Baltimore, MD: Johns Hopkins University Press, 1973.

Wilcox, John T. "Nature as Demonic in Thomson's Defense of Abortion." In *The Ethics of Abortion: Pro-Life Vs. Pro-Choice*, edited by Robert M. Baird and Stuart E. Rosenbaum, 212–225. Buffalo, NY: Prometheus Books, 1993.

Wildes, Kevin Wm. "The Priesthood of Bioethics and the Return of Casuistry." *Journal of Medicine and Philosophy* 18, no. 1 (1993): 33–49.

Wright, Will. *Six Guns and Society: A Structural Study of the Western*. Berkeley, CA: University of California Press, 2008.

Zaner, Richard M. *Ethics and the Clinical Encounter*. Englewood Cliffs, NJ: Prentice Hall, 1988.

———. "Experience and Moral Life: A Phenomenological Approach to Bioethics." In *A Matter of Principles?: Ferment in U.S. Bioethics*, edited by E. R. DuBose, R. P. Hamel, and L. J. O'Connel, 211–239. Valley Forge, PA: Trinity, 1994.

———. *Troubled Voices: Stories of Ethics and Illness*. Cleveland, OH: Pilgrim Press, 1993.

Zarefsky, David. "Presidential Rhetoric and the Power of Definition." *Presidential Studies Quarterly* 34, no. 3 (2004): 607–619.

Zoloth, Laurie. *Health Care and the Ethics of Encounter: A Jewish Discussion of Social Justice*. Chapel Hill, NC: University of North Carolina Press, 1999.

Zussman, Robert. *Intensive Care: Medical Ethics and the Medical Profession*. Chicago, IL: University of Chicago Press, 1994.

Index

About the Author

Tod S. Chambers teaches at Northwestern University's Feinberg School of Medicine in Chicago, IL. His prior book was *The Fiction of Bioethics*.